FOOD BEHAVIOR
WHY WE EAT WHAT WE EAT
Second Edition

Sarah Colby, Editor and Coauthor
East Carolina University

Coauthors
Adrienne A. White, Jennifer R. Walsh, Karla Shelnutt,
David Janicke, Rafael Pérez-Escamilla,
Angela Bermúdez-Millán, Nicole Darmon,
Pablo Monsivais, Melissa Nelson Laska, Jerica M. Berge,
George L. Blackburn, Michael Wheeler,
David Himmelgreen, Nurgül Fitzgerald, Susan Gabriel,
Carol Byrd-Bredbener, Virginia (Ginger) Quick

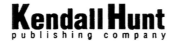

Kendall Hunt
publishing company

Cover image © Shutterstock, Inc.

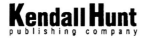

www.kendallhunt.com
Send all inquiries to:
4050 Westmark Drive
Dubuque, IA 52004-1840

Printed in the United States of America
10 9 8 7 6 5 4 3 2

CONTENTS

<u>DEDICATION</u>

This work is dedicated to the family and loved ones of all of the coauthors. Without your love and support, none of us could make it in this crazy little world called academia.

This work is also dedicated to all of the students.
We hope that this book helps you to think about your world
a little differently and someday may help you make someone else's
life a little healthier because you read this.

About the Authors

Jerica Berge, PhD, LMFT

Dr. Berge is an Assistant Professor and behavioral health provider at the University of Minnesota Medical School in the Department of Family Medicine and Community Health. She received her PhD in marriage and family therapy from the University of Minnesota with a minor in public health. Dr. Berge's research interests include family/home environment predictors of child and adolescent obesity, reducing health disparities through community engagement and participatory action research, resiliency of children with chronic illnesses, and clinical effectiveness of family therapy in reducing biopsychosocial problems in youth. Dr. Berge's current research focus is on utilizing relational influences to combat childhood obesity. She is currently on a NIH K-12 award, career development award, to investigate risk and protective factors of childhood obesity in the home environment.

Angela Bermúdez-Millán, PhD, MPH

Dr. Bermúdez-Millán specializes in the area of community nutrition with a strong interest on maternal and child health among minority groups. Her current research interests are on prenatal nutrition, prenatal weight gain and birth outcomes among Latinas. She is currently working as the Coordinator of the Community Connections Core for the Connecticut Center for Eliminating Health Disparities among Latinos (CEHDL), interpreting relevant health disparity information for the community, capturing community perspective on health disparities for interpretation in the world of research, and evaluating community based best-practice solutions to health disparities.

George L. Blackburn, M.D., PhD

Dr. Blackburn is the S. Daniel Abraham Associate Professor of Nutrition and the Associate Director of Nutrition, Division of Nutrition at Harvard Medical School. He is the Chief of the Nutritional/Metabolism Laboratory and Director of the Center for the Study of Nutrition Medicine, which are affiliated with the Beth Israel Deaconess Medical Center in Boston, Massachusetts. In these roles, he is at the forefront of innovations in clinical care, scholarship, mentorship, and education in surgical/medical nutrition and obesity research. His research includes the role of fatty acids and proteins on energy biochemistry, the nutrient effects of bioactive components on cellular and molecular function, and the metabolic correlates of weight loss following surgical treatment of obesity. Recent efforts center on the development and dissemination of best practices in both surgical and non-surgical interventions for the treatment of obesity and obesity-related disease. As part of CSNM's mission to prevent and treat severe obesity, they have launched a novel scientific approach to exercise medicine for weight loss surgery patients. In an ongoing effort to understand the science of healthy living, the CSNM is working with neuroscientists to pioneer research into the neurocognitive correlates of diet and physical activity patterns in lean and obese subjects. Dr. Blackburn received his medical degree from the University of Kansas and completed his internship and residency at Boston City Hospital, Harvard Medical School. He obtained his doctorate in nutritional biochemistry from Massachusetts Institute of Technology. He has trained over 100 fellows in applied and clinical nutrition and has published widely on various aspects of nutrition, medicine, and metabolism, with over 400 publications to date.

Carol Byrd-Bredbenner, PhD, RD, FADA

Dr. Byrd-Bredbenner received her doctorate from Pennsylvania State University. Currently, she is Professor of Nutrition in the Nutritional Sciences Department at Rutgers, The State University of New Jersey. She teaches a wide range of undergraduate and graduate nutrition courses. Her research interests focus on investigating environmental factors that affect dietary choices and health outcomes. Dr. Byrd-Bredbenner has authored numerous nutrition texts, journal articles, and computer software packages. She has received teaching awards from the American Dietetic Association, Society for Nutrition Education, and U.S. Department of Agriculture. In 2007, she received the American Dietetic Association's

Anita Owen Award for Innovative Nutrition Education Programs. She also was a Fellow of the United Nations, World Health Organization at the WHO Collaborating Center for Nutrition Education, University of Athens, Greece.

Sarah Colby, PhD, RD

Dr. Colby received her Bachelor of Science at Florida State University, her Master of Health Science at Western Carolina University and her doctorate at the University of North Carolina at Greensboro. She has worked clinically as a registered dietitian at the Cherokee Reservation hospital and also as a renal dietitian. Dr. Colby also worked with the USDA agricultural research services as a nutrition research scientist. She is currently an Assistant Professor of Nutrition in the Nutrition and Dietetics Department at East Carolina University. Dr. Colby is a behavioral researcher with an obesity prevention focus. She has experience with preschool populations, young adults, nutrition education, participatory action research, Latino and Native American populations, food security, and marketing.

Nicole Darmon, PhD

Dr. Darmon works as an Epidemiologist at the Human Nutrition Research Unit of the INSERM (French National Research Institute of Health and Medicine) and the INRA (National Research Institute on Agronomy) in Marseille, France. She holds an Engineering Degree in Industrial Food Biochemistry and a Ph.D. degree in Human Nutrition. She has conducted nutritional surveys in vulnerable populations, such as homeless and food aid recipients, and she has developed innovative approaches to study the impact of cost constraints on food choices. Based on population diet modeling, she has studied the feasibility of nutritional recommendations, their cost, and their implications in terms of food choices. She is currently developing new tools to increase the quality of individual diets and to assess the nutritional quality of individual foods and their contribution to healthy diets. Dr. Darmon has published over 60 papers in nutrition and public health peer-reviewed journals. As an expert of food poverty and nutrition in industrialized countries and as an expert of diet optimization and nutrient profiling approaches, she has been involved in the definition of the main nutrition prevention and education programmes in France and in several European expert committees.

Nurgül Fitzgerald, PhD, MS, RD

Dr. Fitzgerald is an Assistant Professor in the Department of Nutritional Sciences at Rutgers, The State University of New Jersey. Her work focuses on obesity and diabetes prevention, healthy lifestyle promotion, minority health, and nutritional epidemiology. She uses multifaceted culture- and literacy-appropriate approaches that address individual, family, community, and policy level determinants of health with a special emphasis on socioeconomic factors and food insecurity. She is involved in studies such as building community capacity through peer training, state-wide wellness promotion, and urban farmer's market initiatives. She has taken many leadership roles in various public and professional organizations such as the Society for Nutrition Education, American Society for Nutrition, New Jersey Diabetes Council, Primary Prevention Task Force, and the State Partnership for Nutrition, Physical Activity, and Obesity. She is on the Editorial Board of the Journal of the Nutrition Education and Behavior and teaches graduate and undergraduate level courses.

Susan Gabriel, MS

Susan Gabriel is Associate Director of Evidence-based Medicine, Specialty Medicines Division, at Novartis Pharmaceuticals. She has 20+ years of experience in Marketing Research, spanning multiple industries that include consumer packaged goods, medical devices, and pharmaceuticals. Susan holds a Bachelor of Science degree in Nutritional Sciences, a Master of Science degree in Human Nutrition, and at the time of this publication, pursuing a doctoral degree in Nutritional Sciences at Rutgers, The State University of New Jersey.

David A. Himmelgreen, PhD

Dr. Himmelgreen is an associate professor in the Department of Anthropology at the University of South Florida. His areas of specialization include nutritional anthropology, nutritional assessment, program evaluation and development. Currently, Dr. Himmelgreen is doing NSF funded research on globalization and nutritional health in Costa Rica and on food insecurity and HIV/AIDS in Lesotho, Southern Africa. He has also conducted research on dietary acculturation among Latinos living in the US. Dr. Himmelgreen is an Associate Editor for Ecology of Food and Nutrition and General Editor of the NAPA Bulletin (to be renamed the Annals of Practicing Anthropology).

David M. Janicke, PhD

Dr. Janicke is an Associate Professor in the Department of Clinical and Health Psychology in the College of Public Health and Health Professions at the University of Florida. He received his doctorate in Clinical Psychology from Virginia Polytechnic Institute and State University in 2001. He has over 35 peer reviewed journal publications and book chapters. His primary research and clinical interests are in the area of pediatric obesity, most notably; (a) treatment of pediatric obesity; (b) factors that impact psychosocial functioning in overweight and obese children; (c) the impact of weight status and psychosocial functioning on pediatric health care expenditures; and (d) the translation and dissemination of treatments to community settings. He is currently the primary investigator on a 4.5 year grant funded by NIDDK examining the impact of community-based weight management programs for children and their families in under-served rural communities. Dr. Janicke is on the Editorial Board for the Journal of Pediatric Psychology, and is currently the Associate Editor for a special issue on Rural Health in Pediatric Populations.

Melissa Nelson Laska, PhD, RD

Dr. Laska is a nutritionist and epidemiologist whose primary research interests are in the areas of obesity prevention and nutrition promotion during the emerging adult years (i.e., 18-25). Overall, her research examines contextual, social and behavioral determinants of body weight among childhood, adolescence and young adulthood. Dr. Laska is an Assistant Professor in the Division of Epidemiology and Community Health at the University of Minnesota's School of Public Health. Dr. Laska also serves as a Faculty Research Associate for Healthy Eating Research, a national program of the Robert Wood Johnson Foundation. She received her PhD in Nutrition, with a minor in Epidemiology, from the University of North Carolina at Chapel Hill,as well as a BS with honors in Nutritional Science from Cornell University. Dr. Laska completed her dietetic internship with Vanderbilt University Medical Center and is certified as a Registered Dietitian.

Pablo Monsivais, PhD, MPH

Dr. Monsivais is an investigator at the Center for Public Health Nutrition at the University of Washington's School of Public Health. His research examines the psychological social and demographic factors that influence dietary patterns and diet quality. Prior to his current position, Dr. Monsivais was a senior fellow in behavioral sciences at the UW and a Wellcome Trust research fellow in physiology at University College London.

Rafael Pérez-Escamilla, PhD

Dr. Pérez-Escamilla specializes in domestic and international community nutrition and health disparities. He is a professor of epidemiology and public health at the Yale School of Public Health where he also directs the Office of Community Health. He is founding director and principal investigator of the Connecticut NIH EXPORT Center for Eliminating Health Disparities among Latinos (CEHDL). He also co-founded and led for 15 years, the SNAP-Ed Connecticut Hispanic Family Nutrition Program in full partnership with the Hispanic Health Council in Hartford, Connecticut. For over two decades Dr. Pérez-Escamilla has conducted maternal-child nutrition and food security research in the USA, Latin America and the Caribbean, South America, and West Africa. He has published over 100 research articles and over 250 research abstracts and book chapters. He has been the principal mentor of 40 graduate students and postdoctoral researchers from all over the world. He is a member of the 2010 USA Dietary Guidelines Advisory Committee and an advisory board member of the Pan American Health and Education Foundation. He has been a senior scientific advisor to maternal-child health programs funded by prestigious international agencies including USAID, UNICEF, the World Health Organization, UNDP, and the World Bank.

Karla P. Shelnutt, PhD, RD

Dr. Shelnutt is an Assistant Professor and Extension Nutrition Specialist in the Department of Family, Youth and Community Sciences, University of Florida, Gainesville, Florida. Dr. Shelnutt received a BS in Food Science and Human Nutrition from the University of Florida, an MS in Clinical Nutrition from the University of Alabama at Birmingham where she also completed her dietetic internship, and a PhD in Food Science and Human Nutrition from the University of Florida. Dr. Shelnutt teaches undergraduate nutrition courses in the Food Science and Human Nutrition Department and provides leadership for an Extension program that focuses on lifestyle nutrition and health issues, primarily addressing obesity prevention in children, adolescents, and young adults.

Virginia Quick, RD

Virginia Quick is a doctoral candidate in the Nutritional Sciences Department at Rutgers University. She holds a bachelor's degree in Nutritional Sciences at Rutgers University and currently is pursuing her PhD at Rutgers University. She is a licensed registered dietitian and works part-time as an Outpatient Prenatal Nutritionist in the Women's Health Clinic at Saint Peters University Hospital in New Brunswick, NJ. Her research interests include body image, media, eating disorders, food advertisements directed to children, obesity prevention and food safety education. Ms. Quick also supervises the Nutrition Advocate group on campus that is run through Rutgers University Health Services, overseeing and mentoring 40 undergraduate nutrition students. She is a proud member of the American Dietetic Association, Academy of Eating Disorders, Binge Eating Disorders Association, and Kappa Omicron Nu.

Jennifer R. Walsh, MS, RD

Jennifer R. Walsh is a doctoral candidate in the Department of Food Science and Human Nutrition at the University of Maine. She received her MS in Human Nutrition from the University of Maine in 2006 and became a Registered Dietitian in 2007. Her research focus is community nutrition education and obesity prevention. She is on the Board of the Maine Nutrition Council and holds membership in the American Dietetic Association, Society of Nutrition Education (SNE), and Kappa Omicron Nu.

Michael Wheeler, PhD

Dr. Wheeler is an Associate Professor of Nutrition at East Carolina University. He received his graduate training at UNC with the late Dr. Ronald Thurman, who pioneered the field of alcoholic liver disease with the use of transgenic and knockout mice strains in an intragastric feeding model. As a post-doctoral fellow, he worked with Drs. Jude Samulski and David Brenner, on developing techniques for recombinant gene therapy approach for the treatment of chronic liver diseases. Dr. Wheeler's research has focused on the role of key immune cells in the progression of metabolic diseases, specifically non-alcoholic fatty liver disease, metabolic syndrome, insulin resistance and obesity. His lab has studied how immune cells such as macrophages and liver T cells promote or regulate these various disease states. Interestingly, his works has demonstrated that not only does the immune response contribute to the widely accepted inflammatory response associated with fat accumulation, but also plays a central role in regulating fat metabolism. The associations among the immune response, metabolism, and chronic liver disease may lie at the heart of the initiation of other peripheral tissue pathologies such as obesity and diabetes. Importantly, Dr. Wheeler's lab has developed a number of animal models and genetic mapping techniques and routinely uses standard techniques in molecular and cellular biology to address these and other important questions.

Adrienne White, PhD, RD

Dr. White is a Professor of Human Nutrition at the University of Maine. She received her PhD from the University of Tennessee in 1988 and became a Registered Dietitian in 1989. Since 1997, she has directed the Dietetic Internship, which is integrated with the graduate program. Besides teaching courses for graduate interns, she teaches the undergraduate capstone course, Community Nutrition. Her research is developing, implementing and evaluating theory-based nutrition education interventions. She has been part of a multi-state research team since 1995. She holds membership in the American Dietetic Association, the Society of Nutrition Education (SNE) and the American Association of Family and Consumer Sciences. She is on the Board of SNE, the Maine Dietetic Association, and the Maine Association of Family and Consumer Sciences. In 2007 she received the Mid Career Achievement Award and in 2008 the Helen Dunning Award of Excellence in Nutrition Education, both given by SNE.

FOREWORD

Food. What does that word mean to you? What does that word mean to a starving child in an underdeveloped country? What does that word mean to the CEO of a multimillion-dollar restaurant company? How can one thing have such an incredible impact on our lives? The importance of food is indisputable. At a basic level without food we die. Without adequate food, we get diseases such as scurvy, rickets, or beriberi. With an unbalanced diet people may develop obesity, diabetes, cancer, or heart disease. Food is also an emotional part of our lives. It is important part of ceremonies and traditions such as weddings, funerals, birthdays, Easter, Christmas, and Thanksgiving.

This book is intended to make you think about the factors that influence dietary behaviors. These factors include environmental, economic, cultural, interpersonal, and physiological influences. Occasionally these factors influence behaviors independently, but more often, they influence behaviors through a series of complex interactions. The interactions of these five factors explored in this book are the basis of *The Ecological Model of Food Behavior.*

Chapter 1

Barriers and Food Behavior

Jennifer R. Walsh and Adrienne A. White

Goal: This chapter is an introduction to barriers that prevent people from making healthful food choices and engaging in physical activity.

Objectives: After completing this chapter, you should be able to:

1. Describe barriers to eating healthful foods.
2. Describe barriers to engaging in physical activity.
3. Identify barriers of specific population groups to achieving a healthful diet and engaging in physical activity.
4. Identify how barriers fit in *The Ecological Model of Food Behavior*.

Have you ever been asked to make a choice between French fries or a side salad? Which one did you choose? Do you know why you made that choice? Could it be because the portion for the fries was larger than the salad? Maybe you thought one of the choices was the best way to complement the rest of your meal? Was there peer pressure to choose one or the other? Was your choice influenced by a commercial or maybe an advertisement in a magazine? Do you like the taste of one more than the other?

How about your choice for exercise? Are you more likely to go bowling or skiing? Is your choice influenced by having the skills or the right equipment? Do you only exercise with friends?

There are many determinants that affect our eating and activity choices. The determinants can be internal or external influences. Choices can be influenced by personal attributes like our values and knowledge but also external factors like accessibility of certain foods or recreation areas.

Over the past few decades our society has changed in ways that affect our choices. Grocery stores offer more items than ever, with about 45,000 items available on average in a store (Food Marketing Institute 2006). Convenience stores, restaurants and other food outlets are more prevalent than in the past (Schulter and Lee 1999; Jekanowski 1999). Americans are choosing to eat out more which is a concern since restaurant foods are often associated with higher fat, calories, sodium and lower fiber foods than home-prepared meals (Glanz, Sallis et al. 2005; Popkin, Duffey et al. 2005; Kant, Graubard 2004; Ma, Bertone et al. 2003; Guthrie, Lin et al. 2002). Over the past 30 years, portion sizes have also grown (Nielson and Popkin 2003; Rolls, Morris et al. 2002). In addition to these food changes, we live in a society in which many jobs depend upon a person being sedentary for more than 8 hours a day. Leisure time in America often includes screen time whether it is with a computer, television, or video game. With all these changes, it makes sense that we might try to understand how our choices are shaped each day.

Through this text you will examine influences on your food and physical activity choices. Influences that can be categorized as environmental (availability and marketing), economic (income), interpersonal (how family and friends interact), cultural (acculturation and traditional foods), and physiological factors (disease and genetics) are all part of *The Ecological Model of Food Behavior* (Figure 1). Through the chapters you will have the opportunity to learn and think about the role of these influences on food choice, hunger, and satiety. Practical applications for using *The Ecological Model of Food Behavior* for health program planning will be presented.

Figure 1: The Ecological Model of Food Behavior

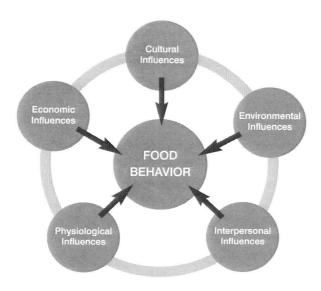

ENERGY BALANCE

All of the choices we make related to eating and physical activity have physiological effects, positive or negative, on our health. Obesity is a result of many choices, made over an extended amount of time, resulting in energy imbalance. Food intake and physical activity make up the key behavior for balancing energy in the body. Through food intake we acquire energy in the form of calories for our body to use and physical activity is a way to expend energy. When the calories taken in are equal to the calories used in a day, weight will remain stable. When more calories are eaten than used, weight is gained. When fewer calories are eaten than used in a day, weight is lost. This balancing act is the reason why our choices related to eating and physical activity are so important and, consequently, a major determinant of body weight.

DIETARY RECOMMENDATIONS

In the Dietary Guidelines for Americans 2005 (Dietary Guidelines for Americans, 2005), recommendations for food intake are based on consuming 2000 calories per day. General guidelines include 2 cups of fruit, 2.5 cups of vegetables, 3 or more ounce-equivalents of whole grain foods, and 3 cups of fat-free or low-fat milk products per day. To reduce chronic disease risk, adults are recommended to engage in at least 30 minutes of moderate intensity physical activity most days of the week. To manage body weight, adults should engage in 60 minutes of moderate to vigorous intensity physical activity on most days of the week. Recommendations vary for some population groups and life stages, especially for older adults and children.

HEALTH BENEFITS

Many Americans recognize the link between food and health and have a general idea of what comprises a healthful diet and active lifestyle. What we eat directly influences our ability to fight infection to prevent illness (morbidity) related to communicable disease, avoid or manage chronic diseases like type 2 diabetes and cardiovascular disease, improve emotional well being, improve appearance, improve the quality of our life, and postpone death (mortality). Thus, many people try to improve their dietary intake and activity to maximize health. If people have this knowledge then why are healthful eating and physical activity recommendations not met by many Americans?

Barriers to making choices for maintaining or achieving a healthful lifestyle prevent people from meeting recommendations for eating healthfully and engaging in physical activity. In this chapter, these barriers and how they are affected by mediating factors like life stage, sex, income, and ethnicity will be discussed. You will also identify how these barriers fit within *The Ecological Model of Food Behavior* and how to address barriers for health promotion programming. Barriers may exist within one factor of the model or through complex interactions where factors of the model overlap.

For example, limited healthful food availability can be an interaction of economic and environmental factors.

HEALTHFUL FOOD BARRIERS

Factors like unpleasant taste, lack of availability of healthful foods, cost, inconvenience, or poor health status can be perceived as barriers to making choices for a healthful lifestyle for most people (Connors, Bisogni et al. 2001; Glanz, Basil et al. 1998). Other barriers may be specific to individual population groups. Through this chapter you will see how barriers may be of greater concern for some population groups than others.

Food insecurity is "a household-level economic and social condition of limited or uncertain access to adequate food" (Economic Research Service/United States Department of Agriculture 2006). For many people food insecurity is a barrier to healthful eating, especially those with low incomes or low socioeconomic status. It is often argued that it is the perception of the cost, not the actual cost that is the barrier to purchasing healthful foods or eating a healthful diet. This stance may vary based on how healthful foods are defined. Foods that are energy-dense (high in calories) are often not as nutrient-dense as foods low in calories, like fruits and vegetables (Andrieu, Darmon et al. 2006). These energy-dense foods are typically less expensive and less likely to be affected by inflation than lower calorie, more nutrient-dense foods (Darmon and Drewnowski 2008; Monsivais and Drewnowski 2007; Andrieu, Darmon et al. 2006). To demonstrate the barrier of food cost, researchers have found that when healthful foods and beverages are subsidized people are more likely to choose them (Brown and Tammineni 2009; Michels, Bloom et al. 2008).

Healthful food inaccessibility and lack of close proximity to supermarkets have been associated with lower dietary quality (Franco, Diez-Roux et al. 2009; Bodor, Rose et al. 2007; Laraia and Siega-Riz et al. 2004). Food environments have been examined in rural and urban communities. In rural neighborhoods healthful food options like low-fat dairy, apples, high fiber bread, and eggs are more available in supermarkets or groceries than in convenience stores (Liese, Weis et al. 2007). Not surprisingly, there is a negative correlation between the distance to a supermarket and population density (Sharkey and Horel 2008; Liese, Weis et al. 2007). Furthermore, healthful food options in rural convenience stores are likely to be priced higher than those in larger food stores, creating an interaction among economic and environmental factors (Liese, Weis et al. 2007). Other examples of this interaction are that poor neighborhoods versus wealthier neighborhoods have more fast food restaurants (Simon, Kwan et al. 2008; Morland, Wing et al. 2002), less stores with healthful options (Horowitz and Colson 2004), and limited transportation, all characteristics that limit access to healthful foods (Morland, Wing et al. 2002).

Healthful Food Barriers and Life Stages

Older Adults

Food choices for the older adults are largely influenced by health status which may necessitate a special diet. Poor dentition is often associated with low-income or minority elders and is a predictor of poor dietary quality (Hendrix, Fischer et al. 2008; Nowjack-Raymer and Sheiham 2007). Similarly, chewing and digestive problems are barriers to eating healthful foods, especially fruits and vegetables. Limited mobility inhibits some elders from being able to food shop for themselves, a barrier to having preferred foods available. Other physiological barriers are inability of self-feeding and changing taste perceptions (Locher, Ritchie et al. 2009; Hendrix, Fischer et al. 2008). Not having people with whom to eat can be an interpersonal barrier for elders. Environmental barriers include grocery stores not having preferred items, lack of storage space, transportation problems, and limited cooking equipment or facilities (Locher, Ritchie et al. 2009; Hendrix, Fischer 2008).

Adults

Most research about healthful eating barriers of adults has been conducted with low-income women. Perceived high cost of healthful foods, especially fruits and vegetables, and lack of time are barriers for low-income adults (Dammann and Smith 2009; Yeh, Ickes et al. 2008). Economic constraints limit food budgets (Chang, Nitzke et al. 2008; Eikenberry and Smith 2004). Without employment or the use of federal assistance programs like the Supplemental Nutrition Assistance Program and Woman, Infants, Children, low-income women are less likely to purchase healthful foods (Dammann and Smith 2009). Time is an issue for women that varies based on employment, and marital and parenting status with convenience ultimately determining many food choices (Jilcott, Larai et al. 2009; Ainsworth, Wilcox et al. 2003).

Interpersonal barriers for adults, to making healthful eating choices, include negative influences of co-workers and family members, especially spouses and children (Jilcott, Laraia et al. 2009; Yeh, Ickes et al. 2008). Household members who are responsible for meal preparation may be influenced by family preferences rather than preparing foods with health as a priority (Dammann and Smith 2009; Chang, Nitzke et al. 2008; Chang, Baumann et al. 2005; Eikenberry and Smith 2004).

The location and layout of a store and product quality and price can be environmental barriers to low-income adults purchasing fruits and vegetables (Webber, Sobal et al. 2010). Limited transportation and number of grocery stores inhibit adults from shopping for affordable healthful foods (Dammann and Smith 2009; Yeh, Ickes, Lowenstein et al. 2008; Eikenberry and Smith 2004). Lack of facilities for food storage, preparation, and dining and lack of structure for mealtimes can all be barriers to eating healthful foods in the home environment (Dammann and Smith 2009).

Young Adults

Young adults are in a time of transition during which lifestyle habits are established (Arnett 2001, 1998, 1997). Maintaining a social life is a priority and may be an interpersonal barrier to making healthful eating choices (Greaney, Lees et al. 2009). Examples of these barriers are eating with friends who choose less healthful foods or eating when not hungry, but just to be with peers. College students have reported that it is their friends, not their family, who influence their eating choices (Strong, Parks et al. 2008). Barriers of fruit and vegetable intake for males are lack of food preparation skills and limited access at home due to spoilage (Walsh,

White et al. 2009). Having easy accessibility to unhealthful food and fast food restaurants can make healthful eating difficult. Taste and temptation are both physiological barriers to eating healthful foods that have been reported by young adults (Walsh, White et al. 2009).

Adolescents

Barriers for adolescents to eat healthful foods include availability, convenience, lack of time, cost, media, a low sense of urgency regarding health issues, social norms, familial and cultural expectations/influences, food appeal, hunger and food cravings (Shepherd, Harden et al. 2005; Spear 2002; Story, Neumark-Sztainer et al. 2002; Croll, Neumark-Sztainer 2001; Neumark-Sztainer, Story et al. 1999; Adams 1997). Healthful eating is often associated with foods at home while less healthful eating behavior is identified with peers (Adams 1997). Furthermore, the general social acceptance of unhealthful eating is a barrier (Adams 1997; Evans 1995). Not having regular family meals has been determined to limit healthful eating behavior and adolescents who do not partake in food preparation may have higher-fat diets and low fruit and vegetable intake (Larson, Story et al. 2006; Neumark-Sztainer, Wall et al. 2003; Neumark-Sztainer, Hannan et al. 2003; Adams 1997).

Environmental barriers to healthful choices for adolescents are access to unhealthful food at school and convenience stores (Bauer, Yang et al. 2004; Adams 1997). Home availability of fruits and vegetables is a strong determinant of intake and can be related to social support, family meal patterns, food security, and socioeconomic status (Neumark-Sztainer, Wall et al. 2003). Adolescents and children from food insecure households may eat less healthful foods, especially fruit and vegetables (Lorson, Melgar-Quinonez et al. 2009).

Children

Parents and primary caregivers are the greatest influences on the choices children make and their fruit and vegetable intake is related to their parents' or primary care givers' ability to prepare and serve these foods (Hildebrand and Betts 2009; Patrick and Nicklas 2005; Benton 2004). Lack of support from family members, child preference, time constraint, convenience and difficulty changing habits are barriers reported by parents to providing children with a healthful diet, limiting fast foods (Sonneville, LaPelle et al. 2009; Hart, Herriot et al. 2003). Parents have reported the school environment, negative food role models, cost, and peer influences to be barriers to their children achieving and maintaining healthful diets (Hart, Herriot et al. 2003). Children with mothers who work outside the home may eat more meals outside the home each week than children with stay-at-home mothers (Siwik and Senf 2006). Television viewing has also been associated with poor diet quality due to low fruit and vegetable intake (Wiecha, Peterson et al. 2006; Coon and Goldberg 2001).

HEALTHFUL FOOD BARRIERS AND ETHNICITY

When people immigrate they typically adopt an American diet with more energy-dense, low-nutrient dense foods than their country of origin (Novotny, Williams et al. 2009; Caballero and Popkin 2002). This phenomenon, which coincides with acculturation, has been explored with Hispanic Americans (Dave, Evans et al. 2009; Colby, Morrison et al. 2009; Duffey, Gordon-Larsen 2008; Sundquist and Winkleby 2000), Black Americans (Bennett, Wolin et al. 2007), and Asian Indians (Mahadevan and Blair 2009). As a result of acculturation, low healthful food availability, traditional food displacement, and high food cost can decrease diet quality (Colby, Morrison et al. 2009). In addition to acculturation, place of birth and age at arrival in the United States may influence food choices (Novotny, Williams et al. 2009).

African Americans

African Americans have reported that barriers to healthful eating involve complex interactions between social and cultural factors (Galasso, Amend et al. 2005; Fitzgibbon and Stolley 2004; James 2004). Attitudes related to food choices are often passed down from generation to generation (Peters, Aroian et al. 2006). Some African Americans feel that eating the recommended diet would require them to desert part of their cultural heritage and conform to practices of the dominant culture (James 2004). Additionally, there are social/cultural symbols associated with certain foods (James 2004). African American women may feel cultural pressure to prepare traditional high-fat foods and an expectation to make large amounts of food for social gatherings (Barnes, Goodrick et al. 2007; Blixen, Singh et al. 2006). There is a lack of social support from friends and significant others to eat healthful foods (Pawlak and Colby 2009). Taste of healthful foods is a physiological barrier for African Americans (Galasso, Amend et al. 2005; James 2004).

African Americans may be more likely to consume fruits and vegetables if they have access to a supermarket than small neighborhood stores (Zenk, Schulz et al. 2005). In many predominately African American neighborhoods there are primarily small grocery stores, with high-fat, energy-dense foods, few grocery stores with fresh produce, and many fast food restaurants (Fitzgibbon and Stolley 2004; Plescia and Groblewski 2004).

Hispanic Americans

Hispanic Americans report time as the primary barrier to eating a healthful diet and engaging in physical activity (Chatterjee, Blakely et al. 2005). Additionally, lack of family support, fewer grocery stores carrying recommended health items, and cost were also reported to be barriers to healthful eating (Albarran, Ballesteros et al. 2005; Horowitz, Colson et al. 2004; Wen, Parchman et al. 2004). Although traditional foods may be available, they are displaced by the abundance of high-fat, high-sugar, processed and fast foods (Colby, Morrison et al. 2009). Food choices may be associated with being part of an Hispanic community where traditional foods like corn, tomatoes, chili peppers and legumes dominate (Reyes-Ortiz, Ju et al. 2009).

Among ethnic groups, Hispanics are more likely to eat out, especially women eating lunch during the work day (Siwik and Senf 2006). Limited English proficiency may affect Hispanics willingness to seek out resources and advice about diet and activity (Lopez-Quintero, Berry et al. 2009). In traditional Hispanic families in which the female is the sole meal decision-maker, females are more likely to report less healthful eating barriers than in families where the male and female share meal decision-making (Arredondo, Elder et al. 2006).

Children who are more acculturated or in food insecure households may have low fruit and vegetable intake (Dave, Evans et al. 2009). Hispanic families, especially the elders, may be less likely to encourage healthful eating habits for weight management in children, since it is acceptable to be fat (Sonneville, LaPelle et al. 2009).

Chinese Americans

Environmental, interpersonal physiological and cultural barriers to healthful eating have been reported by Chinese Americans (Liou and Bauer 2007). Social events like eating with friends make choosing healthful food difficult. Although parents are a positive influence for eating healthfully, peers are a negative influence. Environmental barriers include a high number of fast food restaurants with large portion sizes and media promoting processed convenience foods. Another barrier to a healthful diet is the cultural norm of overeating, often encouraged by relatives (Lion and Bauer 2007).

American Indians

Barriers to following dietary recommendations for American Indians include taste, cost, available food quality, and available food selection (Harnack, Sherwood, et al. 1999; Harnack, Story et al. 1999).

Asian Indians

Immigration to the United States by Asian Indians may be associated with decreased intakes of traditional foods (vegetables, lentils, legumes, and grains) and increased intake of easily accessible foods like hamburgers, pizza, and soda (Mahadevan and Blair 2009). Shifts from a vegetarian to a more meat-based diet may occur. Reasons for the changes include lack of time for traditional food preparation and limited availability of spices and ingredients.

Physical Activity Barriers and Life Stages

Older Adults

Health conditions are the primary barrier to achieving recommended levels of physical activity for older adults. In addition to health status, other barriers identified have been the availability and convenience of facilities, physician advice, lack of exercise knowledge, and a lack of belief in the health benefits related to engaging in recommended physical activities (Kearney and McElhone 1999).

Adults

Whereas, the primary barrier to physical activity for older adults is health, the primary barrier to physical activity for middle-aged adults is time. For females, time is often limited due to family and work responsibilities (O'Dougherty, Dallman et al. 2008). Other barriers are lack of social support from friends and family, health status, and fear of injury (O'Dougherty, Dallman et al. 2008; King, Castro et al. 2000; Wilcox, Castro et al. 2000; Scharff, Homan et al. 1999). Economic and environmental barriers to physical activity include cost, lack of available facilities, and concerns of safety (O'Dougherty, Dallman et al. 2008; Popkin, Duffey et al. 2005; Brett, Heimendinger et al. 2002; Zunft, Friebe et al. 1999).

Young Adults

Decreases in physical activity levels are characteristic of the transition from adolescence to young adulthood (Gordon-Larsen, Nelson et al. 2004). Young adults attending college balance school, work and a social life resulting in time being a barrier to physical activity (Greaney, Lees et al. 2009; Walsh, White et al. 2009). Sometimes friends and significant others do not offer support for being physically active and finances are a barrier to use of gym and recreational facilities.

Adolescents

As with young adulthood, physical activity decreases with adolescence (Sallis 2000). Availability of video games, computers and limited access to fitness equipment and fitness facilities negatively affects physical activity for adolescents (Porter, Bean et al. 2010). They also share environmental concerns of unsafe neighborhoods for walking and biking (Porter, Bean et al. 2010; Bauer, Yang et al. 2004). Parent and peer influence, teasing or bullying, and competition can all affect levels of physical activity (Porter, Bean et al. 2010; King, Tergerson et al. 2008; Bauer, Yang et al. 2004).

Children

As with eating, parents and primary caregivers greatly influence the activity level of children. Parents' economic concerns include lack of transportation and cost of exercise resources and organized sports (Sonneville, LaPelle et al. 2009; Hart, Herriot et al. 2003). Similar to other life stages, barriers to physical activity are time constraints, lack of social support, unsafe neighborhoods and limited exercise facilities.

Physical Activity Barriers and Ethnicity

In addition to healthful eating choices, the mediating factor of ethnicity plays a role in engaging in physical activity. Non-Hispanic White Americans report more physical activity during leisure time than Mexican- and African-Americans (Crespo, Smit et al. 2000) and acculturated Hispanic Americans report more physical activity during leisure time than those less acculturated (Crespo, Smit et al. 2001). Additionally, there is a disproportionate amount of high minority communities with limited access to physical activity facilities or resources (Popkin, Duffey et al. 2005).

African Americans

Time and the cost of facilities and exercise are barriers to physical activity for African Americans (Barnes, Goodrick et al. 2007; Nies, Volman et al. 1999). Other negative predictors of physical activity are advanced age, large family size, and low socio-economic status (O'Dougherty, Dallman et al. 2008; Masse and Anderson 2004; Eyler and Vest 2002; Eyler, Brownson et al. 1999). Social norms may also be a barrier because certain physical activities may not be perceived as acceptable or common (Plescia and

Groblewski 2004; Fitzgibbon and Stolley 2004). Environmental barriers include limited access to safe, low crime areas for exercise (Greenberg and Renne 2005; Plescia and Groblewski, 2004; Fitzgibbon and Stolley 2004; King, Castro et al. 2000; Eyler, Baker et al. 1998). Examples of unsafe environmental factors are few sidewalks, inadequate street lighting, and unattended dogs (Ainsworth, Wilcox et al. 2003).

Hispanic Americans

As with African Americans, social norms influence Mexican Americans' physical activity (Colby, Morrison et al. 2009). Mexican Americans may not engage in activities like biking, and traditional forms of activity, like dancing, may not be perceived as socially acceptable in the United States (Colby, Morrison et al. 2009). They have reported reluctance to participate in organized sports due to unfamiliarity and not having other Hispanics involved. Environmental barriers include neighborhoods being unsafe (e.g. sidewalks, physical activity facilities, slope, land use, intersection frequency, and population density) and schools and shopping centers too far away for walking (Chatterjee, Blakely et al. 2005; Rutt and Coleman 2005).

American Indians

Barriers to physical activity in American Indian communities include time, lack of childcare, health problems, and safety concerns (Harnack, Sherwood et al. 1999; Harnack, Story et al. 1999).

OTHER BARRIERS

Has your mood ever determined the choice you made about eating or exercise? If so, it is an intrapersonal influence meaning occurring from inside you. These types of influences include beliefs, attitudes, and feelings and are not part of *The Ecological Model of Food Behavior* because they vary by individual and are influenced by the five factors. Healthful eating intrapersonal barriers may be a perception that meeting recommendations is impossible or just too much trouble (Hendrix, Fischer et al. 2008). Other examples are lack of knowledge, self-control, self-efficacy, food preparation skills, sense of urgency about health, boredom, stress, and laziness (Walsh, White et al. 2009; Pawlak and Colby 2009; Greaney, Lees et al. 2008; Eikenberry and Smith 2004; Chang, Brown et al. 2008; Liou and Bauer 2007; Galasso, Amend et al. 2005; James 2004). Examples of these barriers to being physically active are lack of knowledge, self-efficacy, feeling exhausted, lack of self-confidence, lack of motivation or energy, or not enjoying exercise (Porter, Bean et al. 2010; Sonneville, LaPelle et al. 2009; Kiviniemi and Duangdao 2009; Yeh, Ickes et al. 2008; Chang, Nitzke et al. 2008; O'Dougherty, Dallman et al. 2008; Hendrix, Fischer et al. 2008; King, Castro et al. 2000). In addition to these intrapersonal barriers, time is a barrier that, although mentioned throughout this chapter, is also not part of *The Ecological Model of Food Behavior*.

Barriers and *The Ecological Model of Food Behavior*

The barriers discussed in this chapter fit in *The Ecological Model of Food Behavior*, shown in Figure 2. Concerns of food expense or limited financial resources for food purchases are part of the economic factor. Environmental barriers include the built environment, especially in low-income neighborhoods, or fast food restaurants located near schools. Physiological barriers include the taste of healthful foods and the influence of one's health status. Cultural barriers may be making food choices to maintain cultural roots or because of religious customs. Although these five factors rarely influence behavior in a vacuum independent of one another, the following chapters will help you examine each factor in-depth. By reading this book, you will gain understanding of the multiple and complex factors that influence food behavior.

HEALTH PROGRAM PLANNING

The case is made in this chapter that food choice is primarily dependent on economic, environmental, cultural, interpersonal, and physiological factors that make up *The Ecological Model of Food Behavior*. To respond to the multifactorial, interrelational influences on food behavior, a broad

Figure 2: Barriers and The Ecological Model of Food Behavior

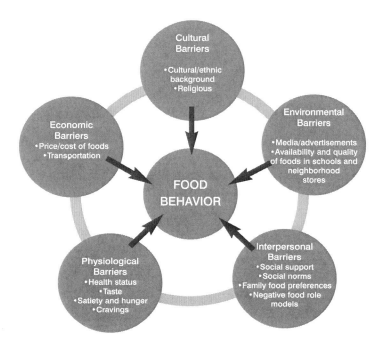

approach for health promotion program planning is needed. Such an approach will demand collaborative efforts across disciplines, community partnerships, environmental supports and policy changes at local, state and national levels.

Fitzgerald and Spaccarotella (2009) identified practical ways for Cooperative Extension professionals to develop and implement programs to promote healthful food choices and physical activity. Their intervention ideas can be applied to others in the public health arena. Using an ecological perspective, as well, they suggested programs to overcome barriers at the intrapersonal; interpersonal; community/institution; and macro/public policy level. They suggested targeting such factors as knowledge, skills and confidence for an intrapersonal level; peer support of the interpersonal level; improving neighborhood safety through community partnerships and policy changes for the community/ institutional level; and establishing partnerships with local restaurants and collaborating with local businesses for worksite wellness for the macro/public policy level. Smith and Morton (2009) recommended strong civic engagement to improve healthful food access by organizations working together to limit barriers through policies, community action, and volunteerism.

When considering population groups, specifically, programs for low-income groups should focus on quick and easy healthful ways to prepare food on a limited budget and identification of inexpensive, convenient healthful foods (Eikenberry and Smith 2004). Programs for children should be targeted to parents and primary caregivers, who should be encouraged to be role models. Cultural implications should be considered when presenting recommendations.

Key Points

1. The five factors that influence food behavior are environmental, economic, cultural, interpersonal, and physiological which form a multifactorial, interrelated model.
2. Barriers to achieving a healthful diet and engaging in physical activity can be categorized under each of the five factors of the model.
3. Barriers to achieving a healthful diet and engaging in physical activity may be associated with life stages and ethnicity.

Nutrition Practice Points

When counseling an individual, it is important to listen to that person's unique set of barriers. Let the individual set his or her own priorities and goals. When an individual has set his or her own diet change goals, it is important for nutrition professionals to consider all five influences of behavior identified in *The Ecological Model of Food Behavior* to anticipate potential barriers the individual may face in trying to reach his or her goals. Although a person can identify many of his or her own barriers, the individual may not be aware of other barriers he or she may encounter. Ask probing questions to determine the current level of social and cultural support for making changes and to assess the influence of the social environment, economic resources, and food availability and preferences on his or her food behavior. Help the individual to address any additional potential barriers identified. By anticipating barriers the person may face, you can help him or her more successfully reach individual diet and activity change goals.

Terminology

Acculturation—The process by which immigrants adopt the attitudes, values, customs, beliefs, and behavior of a new culture.

Barriers—Anything that makes it harder or prevents a person from doing what he or she is trying to do.

Built environment—Everything in the physical environment. This would include sidewalks, grocery stores, outdoor lighting, stop signs, etc.

Intrapersonal—Feelings, attitudes, and beliefs that occur within an individual's own mind.

Nutrient Density—The amount of nutrients a food provides given the amount of calories that food provides. You could eat two meals both providing 400 calories. If one of the meals consisted of whole wheat bread, lean turkey, tomatoes, baby spinach, baby carrots, and skim milk, it would provide more nutrients (be more nutrient-dense) than another meal that also provided 400 calories but consisted only of donuts and soda.

Obesity—Commonly defined by using a body mass index formula (BMI). BMI uses height and weight to estimate body mass (kilograms in weight divided by height in meters squared or kg/m2). BMI is a useful tool when describing populations or an individual's risk compared to a population. Research has shown increased BMI is related to increased risk of developing chronic disease such as diabetes and heart disease. Using BMI alone to describe an individual's body mass or obesity status may be problematic because the BMI formula cannot distinguish between weight of fat mass from weight of muscle mass. A very muscular person may be incorrectly classified by the BMI formula as being overweight or obese. A BMI of 18.5-24.99 indicates a person is normal weight. A BMI of 25-29.9 indicates a person is overweight. A BMI equal to or greater than 30 indicates obesity.

Satiety—Feeling physically full and not hungry after eating.

Self-efficacy—The belief that you would be able to do something if you wanted to do it.

Social Norm—Something that is perceived, accepted, and approved of within a group of people.

ACTIVITY

Write down a specific goal for healthful eating and physical activity to achieve this week. A healthful eating goal may be making at least half your grains whole grains or eating two cups of fruit daily. You may decide to increase the time you spend being physically active or the intensity of an activity. Over the week monitor and log your experiences and what made it easy or difficult to try to achieve your goals. How would you classify each of the influences according to *The Ecological Model of Food Behavior*?

Chapter 2

Obesity in America: A Big Problem

Karla Shelnutt and David Janicke

Goal: This chapter discusses the causes and consequences of obesity.

Objectives: After completing this chapter, you should be able to:

1. Define obesity and describe how it is measured.
2. List potential health consequences of obesity.
3. Discuss potential social and psychological outcomes associated with obesity.

SO WHAT'S THE BIG PROBLEM WITH OBESITY?

Americans have gotten heavier over the past 40 years, leading to a significant increase in the prevalence of obesity. Obesity plays an important role in the development of heart disease, diabetes, and cancer; and thereby contributes to the major causes of death in the United States (Calle, Rodriguez et al. 2003; Berenson 1986; Berenson, McMahan et al. 1980). Obese adults experience a lower quality of life, increased medical expenses, and miss more work than non-obese adults (Finkelstein, Ruhm et al. 2005; Finkelstein, Fiebelkorn et al. 2004; Sturm, Ringel et al. 2004; Bungum, Satterwhite et al. 2003; Fontaine, Redden et al. 2003; Ford, Moriarty et al. 2001; Burton, Chen et al. 1999). Severe obesity can reduce life expectancy by five to twenty years (Fontaine, Redden et al. 2003). With these consequences it is more important than ever to expand our knowledge of the problem and to work together towards finding innovative solutions to address the obesity epidemic.

Defining Obesity

In order to appreciate the magnitude of the negative effects of obesity on health, it is important to understand the problem. Although it is possible to weigh more than predetermined standards (overweight) without being obese, as is the case with athletes who have substantial muscle mass, the classification of obesity refers to a person with excess body fat (National Institutes of Health 1998). There are a variety of methods available to estimate body fat:

1. **Skinfold thickness**: Subcutaneous fat deposits are measured by skinfold thickness. A trained person uses skin calipers to measure triceps, pectoral, abdominal, suprailiac, and thigh skinfold thickness. Measurements are entered into an equation to estimate body density (Jackson, Pollock et al. 1980; Jackson and Pollock 1978), which is then used to calculate body fat.

2. **Waist circumference**: Abdominal fat is associated with a higher risk for certain health problems than fat deposited in other places in the body (National Institutes of Health 1998). Waist circumference is a simple measure of abdominal fat. A tape measure is placed around the abdomen above the hip bones. Women with a waist circumference greater than 35 inches and men with a waist circumference greater than 40 inches have a higher risk for certain diseases than people with a smaller waist circumference (National Institutes of Health 1998).

3. **Bioelectrical impedance analysis** (**BIA**): Impedance of an electrical current passed through the body is used to estimate body fat and lean body mass. Although this method must be performed under controlled conditions to avoid error, it has been validated and is

considered a useful and accurate measure when performed correctly (Segal, Van Loan et al. 1988).

4. **Dual energy x ray absorptiometry** (**DEXA**): Two x-ray energies are used to measure three components of body composition: fat, muscle, and bone mineral density. The subject must lie on a table while the body is scanned. Computer software calculates body composition using x-ray data.

5. **Hydrostatic** (**under water**) **weighing**: Historically considered the "gold standard" of body composition, this method utilizes Archimedes' Principle, which states that the buoyant force on a submerged object is equal to the weight of the fluid displaced. A person with less body fat will weigh more under water than a person with more body fat because fat is less dense than water while fat-free mass is more dense than water. Body density is estimated by determining under water weight and is then used to calculate body fat.

6. **Air displacement** (**Bod Pod**): Instead of using water, body density is estimated by measuring air displacement in a special cylinder. Bod Pod measurements correlate well with DEXA and hydrostatic weighing and is considered an easier method to utilize (Fields, Goran et al. 2002).

7. **Body Mass Index** (**BMI**): The most commonly used indicator of body fatness is BMI, which is a measure of weight based on height, and can be used to determine someone's health risks associated with weight status. BMI is highly correlated to body fatness and is calculated as weight in kilograms divided by height in meters squared. For adults, BMI is not gender specific. Instead, BMI ranges have been established by the World Health Organization (Organization 1998) and the National, Heart, Lung, and Blood Institute (National Institutes of Health 1998) that classify adults as underweight ($\leq$18.5), normal (18.5-24.9), overweight (25-29.9), and obese ($\geq$30). BMI status for children and adolescents aged two to eighteen is classified using gender specific BMI-for-age growth charts available at: http://www.cdc.gov/growthcharts/. Once BMI percentile

is calculated, weight status category is determined using the value in the following table:

Weight Status Category	Percentile Range
Underweight	Less than the 5th percentile
Healthy Weight	5th percentile to less than the 85th percentile
Overweight	85th percentile to less than the 95th percentile
Obese	Equal to or greater than the 95th percentile

Statistics

In the 1970s, only 15 percent of adults were obese. From the 1970s through 2000s the number of obese adults more than doubled to 33.8 percent. An additional 34.2 percent of Americans were also considered overweight, according to National Health and Nutrition Examination Survey (NHANES) data obtained in 2007-2008 (Flegal, Carroll et al. 2010). The percentage of adults categorized as extremely obese (BMI ≥ 40) increased from 0.9 percent in 1960-1962 to 6.2 percent in 2005-2006 (Prevention 2008; Ogden, Carroll et al. 2007;). In the 2000s, over 72 million American adults were obese (Ogden, Carroll et al. 2007). In the late 2000s the increase in obesity appeared to be slowing among women. Flegal et al. reported no significant differences in the prevalence of obesity in women between the analyzed years 1999-2000 and 2007-2008 (33.4% and 35.5%, respectively), even when adjusted for race and ethnicity (Flegal, Carroll et al. 2010). For men there was a significant increase between these years, but when the authors evaluated the years in between they did not find a significant change between 2003-2004, 2005-2006, and 2007-2008. When adjusted for race and ethnic group, there was a significant increase in the prevalence of obesity between 1999-2000 and 2007-2008 in non-Hispanic whites, and non-Hispanic blacks but not in Mexican Americans.

Obesity is no longer a concern only for adults. Between the 1970s and the 2000s the percentage of overweight and obese children and adolescents aged two to nineteen tripled. Estimates from NHANES 2007-2008 of this age group indicated that 14.8 percent of children and adolescents were overweight and 16.9 percent were obese (Ogden, Carroll et al. 2010). Five years old is the mean age for when obesity begins, and obese children are more likely to become obese adults (Salbe, Weyer et al. 2002; Salbe, Weyer et al. 2002; Whitaker, Pepe et al. 1998; Guo, Roche et al. 1994; Serdula, Ivery et al. 1993; Webber, Cresanta et al. 1986).

Disparities

There are disparities in obesity prevalence among different demographic groups. According to NHANES 2007-2008, non-Hispanic black adults had the highest prevalence of obesity (44 percent) followed by Mexican Americans (40 percent), all Hispanics (39 percent) and non-Hispanic whites (32 percent) (Flegal, Carroll et al. 2010). Within racial groups there also were disparities by gender. Non-Hispanic black women consistently had a higher prevalence of obesity than non-Hispanic black men (52.9 percent vs 37.2 percent, respectively, in NHANES 2005-2006 and 49.6 percent vs 37.3 percent, respectively, in NHANES 2007-2008) (Flegal, Carroll et al. 2010; Ogden 2009). A study investigating the potential social factors contributing to the difference in obesity between young black men and women found that parental education was the only factor that modulated risk for obesity between genders (Robinson, Gordon-Larsen et al. 2009).

In children, racial and ethnic differences in the prevalence of obesity also exist. According to data from NHANES 2007-2008, the percentage of obesity and overweight and obesity combined in children two to nineteen years of age was 20 percent and 35.9 percent in non-Hispanic blacks, 20.8 and 38.9 percent in Mexican Americans, 20.9 and 38.2 percent in all Hispanics and 15.3 and 29.3 percent in non-Hispanic whites. Hispanic boys had a significantly higher risk of obesity than non-Hispanic white boys. Non-Hispanic black girls had a significantly higher risk of obesity than non-Hispanic white girls (Ogden, Carroll et al. 2010). The differences among racial groups may be explained by cultural influences on physical activity and family attitudes about food and eating, as well as access to healthy foods and physical activity facilities, which may promote weight gain (Prevention 2009).

Socioeconomic status (SES) also is associated with the risk for obesity with low SES inversely associated with risk for obesity in developed countries, especially in women (McLaren 2007). The effect of family income on obesity risk within races and ethnic groups differs by race. The risk of obesity in children was positively correlated to family income in African American families and inversely correlated in white and Mexican American children (Freedman, Ogden et al. 2007). Among elementary school children, lower SES is associated with being overweight, and the relationship is stronger for girls than boys (Wolfe, Campbell et al. 1994). For children up to eight years of age at baseline in the National Longitudinal Survey of Youth, the six-year incidence of obesity was higher among low-income children, children whose parent(s) had less than a high school education, and African Americans compared to whites or Hispanics (Strauss and Knight 1999).

The Cost of Obesity

Medical expenses in the United States in 2009 related to overweight/obesity were estimated at approximately $79.5 billion dollars. If obesity rates continue to increase at the current rate, 42.8 percent (103 million) of adults will be obese by 2018. This translates into approximately $344 billion dollars projected to be spent on obesity-related healthcare costs in 2018 (Humphries 2009). Data also suggest that adults and children who are obese incur higher healthcare costs than their healthy weight peers (Hampl, Carroll et al. 2007; Thorpe, Florence et al. 2004). Despite the monetary losses, the human cost associated with obesity is even more significant.

Physical Health Risks of Obesity

It was estimated that the average adult gains approximately 1.4 pounds per year (Yanovski, Yanovski et al. 2000); however, weight change of no more than five pounds in one year has been established as defining weight maintenance (St Jeor, Brunner et al. 1997). A BMI greater than 25 has been suggested for use as an "action point for obesity prevention" because of associated increases in health risks (Oh, Shin et al. 2004), although the exact BMI where these health risks begin is controversial (National Institutes of Health 1998). Although the negative impact of obesity on life expectancy varies by race and ethnicity, overall Americans lose one-third to three-fourths of a year of life expectancy due to obesity (Olshansky, Passaro et al. 2005). Currently, many studies indicate that a BMI >25 is related to increased risks and incidence of depression (Johnston, Johnson et al. 2004; Roberts, Deleger et al. 2003), cardiovascular disease (Burke, Beilin et al. 2005; Joshi, Day et al. 2005; Ajani, Lotufo et al. 2004; Jefferys, McCarron et al. 2003; Lamon-Fava, Wilson et al. 1996), stroke (Kurth, Gaziano et al. 2005; Kurth, Gaziano et al. 2002; Rexrode, Hennekens et al. 1997), hypertension (Wilsgaard, Schirmer et al. 2000), dyslipidemia (Brown, Higgins et al. 2000), diabetes (Steyn, Mann et al. 2004; Must, Spadano et al. 1999;), diabetes related cataracts (Weintraub, Willett et al. 2002), chronic kidney disease (Gelber, Kurth et al. 2005), kidney stones (Taylor, Stampfer et al. 2005), end stage renal disease (Hsu, McCulloch et al. 2006), gallstones (Kodama, Kono et al. 1999), cancers and cancer mortality rate (Hou, Ji et al. 2006; Otani, Iwasaki et al. 2005; Jeffreys, Smith et al. 2004; Morimoto, White et al. 2002; Okasha, McCarron et al. 2002; Rodriguez, Calle et al. 2002; Rodriguez, Patel et al. 2001), decreased health-related quality of life (Ford, Moriarty et al. 2001) and mortality (Flegal, Graubard et al. 2006; Flegal, Graubard et al. 2005; Hjartaker, Adami et al. 2005; Flegal, Graubard et al. 2004; Flegal, Williamson et al. 2004; Katzmarzyk, Craig et al. 2002). A recent review of four large studies compared the use of BMI versus other measures of central adiposity (waist circumference, waist-hip ratio, and waist-height ratio) to determine risk for coronary heart disease, diabetes, and all-cause mortality. BMI correlated highly with the other measures and was determined an acceptable measure of risk (Taylor, Ebrahim et al. 2010).

Body Fat Percent

Increased fat mass has also been associated with increased health risks such as cardiovascular disease (CVD) (Katzmarzyk, Gagnon et al. 2001), metabolic syndrome (Zhu, Wang et al. 2003), and increased mortality (Heitmann, Erikson et al. 2000). Increased fat mass alone is a risk factor. Individuals with a normal BMI and a high percent body fat are at increased risk (He, Tan et al. 2001). Increased body fat has been found to be a better indicator of CVD risk than aerobic fitness level (Christou, Gentile et al. 2005). For women, ideal body weight has been suggested to be a body fat percentage less than 30 percent (Hendler, Welle et al. 1995). A percent body fat of 20 percent for men and 30 percent for women is equivalent to a BMI of 25 (Zhu, Wang et al. 2003).

Waist Circumference

Recently, central adiposity has been suggested to be more indicative of health risk than BMI (Zhu, Heshka et al. 2004; Zhu, Wang et al. 2002). Waist circumference is an indicator of central adiposity. Researchers have found data to suggest that individuals below the cut-off points for overweight (BMI < 25) but with increased waist circumference (greater than 32 inches for women and greater than 35 inches for men) have a higher incidence of developing metabolic syndrome (Yeh, Chang et al. 2005). Increased abdominal obesity has been found to be a stronger predictor of insulin insensitivity than fitness level (Racette, Evans et al. 2006). Increased abdominal adiposity is also related to increased risk of developing CVD (Baik, Ascherio et al. 2000) (despite weight status) (Tanaka, Togashi et al. 2002), cancer (Xu, Matthews et al. 2005), arthritis (Janssen and Mark 2006), hypertension (Okosun, Choi et al. 2001; Cox, Whichelow et al. 1997), dyslipidemia (Sattar, Tan et al. 1998), and diabetes (Rosenthal, Jin et al. 2004; al-Asfoor, al-Lawati et al. 1999). Although varying cut-off values have been recommended, a waist circumference greater than 35 inches for women and greater than 40 inches for men has been suggested to identify individuals with increased health risks for hypertension, diabetes, dyslipidemia, and the metabolic syndrome (Janssen, Katzmarzyk et al. 2002).

Psychosocial Risks of Obesity

In addition to the financial impact of obesity related medical costs and human cost measured as reduced life expectancy, the human cost may also be measured in emotional stress and less than optimal psychological functioning.

Obesity is a complex social phenomenon. It is often viewed as associated with some aspect of psychological or emotional distress. Although many studies have tried to find a specific psychological profile associated with obesity, no general profiles have been elucidated. Instead it appears that certain characteristics of obese persons increase their risk for psychological problems (Fabricatore and Wadden 2004). In a review of the literature, Fabricatore and Wadden reported that obese women, extreme obesity, and binge eating increase the risk of suffering from psychological problems such as depression, and that the psychological issues should be addressed before weight loss is attempted (Fabricatore and Wadden 2004).

Obese persons are often stereotyped by others as being lazy, unintelligent, and unsuccessful (Puhl and Heuer 2010). Unfortunately, the propagation of these stereotypes leads to a negative stigma or "weight bias" held by many people, including health professionals who work with obese persons (Bocquier, Verger et al. 2005; Foster, Wadden et al. 2003; Schwartz, Chambliss et al. 2003; Harvey and Hill 2001). Andreyeva et al. examined the change in prevalence of weight bias in Americans over the years and reported a 5 percent increase to 12 percent in all populations except older adults from 1995-1996 to 2004-2006 (Andreyeva, Puhl et al. 2008). Shockingly, this prevalence is equivalent to that of racial and age discrimination yet weight bias lacks the consequences associated with racial and age discrimination (Andreyeva, Puhl et al. 2008). People may blame obese persons for letting themselves gain excessive weight, which may lead to the harmful justification of their stigmatization (Puhl and Heuer 2010). This may in part explain why obese individuals have been discriminated against in the work force. Obese individuals earn less than leaner coworkers do (Puhl and Brownell 2001; Baum and Ford 2004) and are often the target of offensive jokes (Puhl and Heuer 2009; Puhl and Brownell 2006; Puhl and Brownell 2001). More troubling is the stigma associated with obese children. Latner et al. investigated the obesity stigma in children by showing 5th and 6th graders drawings of diverse children (healthy, crutches, wheelchair, missing hand, facial disfigurement, and obese) and asking them to rank the drawings from most to least favorable (Latner and Stunkard 2003). The children ranked the obese child as the least favorable. This study was a replication of the original study from 1961 and showed that the discrimination against the obese child was even greater in 2001. Obese children are often teased and humiliated, which can lead to low self-esteem and possibly struggles later in life for the obese children (Pierce and Wardle 1997).

As more and more Americans are becoming overweight, a positive outcome from the obesity crisis is that more overweight positive role models are appearing in the media. Actors who are considered too thin are getting more negative attention in the press. How does exposure to media images of very thin beautiful people actually impact how the viewers feel about themselves? Does it actually change food and activity patterns? Research has not been able to answer these questions.

Different community groups have different social norms regarding weight. Historically, African American and Latino communities have been more accepting of larger body shapes and have higher body satisfaction than Caucasians (Miller, Gleaves et al. 2000). In many instances, fuller volume figures were considered more attractive than very thin body shapes.

CAN YOU BE FAT AND FIT?

There is a debate over whether a person can be overweight and "fit" or if a lower body weight is an essential component of health. Research has shown that minor, yet clinically significant improvements in glycemic control can be achieved through physical activity that does not result in weight loss (Ibanez, Izquierdo et al. 2005; Miller and Dunstan 2004). Additionally, physical activity without weight reduction has been found to reduce total and visceral fat (Lee, Kuk et al. 2005). According to the results of a review on the effects of physical activity, fitness and body fat on risks for all-cause mortality, cardiovascular mortality and chronic diseases, people with higher BMI but good aerobic fitness have a lower risk for all-cause and cardiovascular mortality than normal weight people with poor fitness levels (Fogelholm 2009) supporting the notion that it is possible to be fat and fit. The authors emphasize that the results may not apply to a BMI greater than 35. Despite these results, others have reported that being fit does not completely reverse the dangers associated with being fat (Stevens, Cai et al. 2002). In their cohort from the Lipid Research Clinics Study, Stevens et al. (Stevens, Cai et al. 2002) reported that the highest levels of fatness and the lowest levels of fitness were associated with an increased all cause and CVD mortality. When comparing fitness between subjects in the lowest four quintiles of BMI (18.7-27.6) to the fifth quintile (27.7-42.6), a significant risk for all-cause mortality was still observed.

It has long been accepted that increased body weight increases bone mass, which could potentially decrease the risk for osteoporosis (Reid, Ames et al. 1992; Reid, Plank et al. 1992). The extra weight from the excess body fat increases the stress on the bone and may promote strength (Zhao, Jiang et al. 2008). On the other hand, too much fat mass may actually be damaging to bone (Zhao, Jiang et al. 2008).

WHAT CAUSES OBESITY?

Obesity is a complex issue that results from multiple factors, including genetics, energy imbalance, environment, and socioeconomic status (Prevention 2009). The major underlying factor contributing to obesity is energy imbalance. Americans are consuming more calories than they are using, which leads to weight gain. This section will focus on factors that lead to excess caloric intake.

Portion Sizes

The increase in portion sizes is one of the problems. The Portion Distortion Quiz from the National Heart Lung and Blood Institute (http://hin.nhlbi.nih.gov/portion) shows consumers how the portion sizes have increased over the years. This is such an important issue for consumers that the Dietary Guidelines for Americans, 2005, includes a paragraph on portion sizes in the weight management chapter. Restaurants offer huge portions so consumers feel like they are getting more food for their money (Activity 2006). Convenience items have also gotten bigger. Young and Nestle compared current portion sizes of various foods to US Department of Agriculture (USDA) and Food and Drug Administration (FDA) standard portion sizes (Young and Nestle 2002). All foods they compared except sliced white bread significantly exceeded the USDA and FDA standard sizes with cookies having the largest surplus at 700 percent. The authors describe the importance of large portion sizes for marketing purposes. They also indicate that additional evidence for increased portion sizes is seen in the lower number of servings specified in identical recipes over the newer editions of the *Joy of Cooking* cookbook as well as the larger cup holders found in cars. Large portion sizes increase caloric intake and may cause people to eat more food. Unfortunately research suggests that people often do not know how to correctly estimate the amount of food that they eat (Activity 2006). Teaching consumers proper portion sizes for when they eat out or at home is an important step in helping to control caloric intake.

Dietary Quality

Although Americans are consuming more calories, the quality of those calories is not high. The Healthy Eating Index (HEI) (Kennedy, Ohls et al. 1995) provides an overall picture of the type and quantity of foods an individual consumes, his or her adherence with specific dietary recommendations, and the variety in the diet. In 2006 the USDA Center for Nutrition Policy and Promotion revised the HEI to compare diets to recommendations from the Dietary Guidelines for Americans, 2005 (Guenther, Krebs-Smith et al. 2006). The individual components evaluated in the HEI-2005 are total fruit, whole fruit, total vegetables, dark green and orange vegetables and legumes, total grains, whole grains, milk, meat and beans, oils, saturated fat, sodium, calories from solid fats, alcoholic beverages, and added sugars. Guenther et al. used the HEI-2005 to evaluate the diet of Americans at two different time points using survey data from the Continuing Survey of Food Intakes by Individuals, 1994-96, and the National Health and Nutrition Examination Survey, 2001-02 (Guenther, Juan et al. 2008). In both surveys all individual component scores were below the maximum score except for total grains and meat and beans. The two lowest scores at both time points were for whole grains and dark green and orange vegetables and legumes. Whole fruit, total vegetables, and whole grains consumption decreased significantly between the two time points. Milk, oils, and sodium increased. Total HEI-2005 scores out of 100 were 58.2 for both surveys, indicating the need for Americans to improve the quality of their diets by choosing more nutrient-dense, high-quality foods. Studies are needed to compare diet quality of Americans since the Dietary Guidelines, 2005, were introduced to determine whether they have had a beneficial impact.

Dietary Diversity

Dietary diversity within and between food groups is not related to total energy, fat, sugar, sodium, or cholesterol intake (Krebs-Smith, Smiciklas-Wright et al. 1987). However, individuals who consume the greatest variety of foods from all food groups have the most adequate nutrient intakes (Kant, Block et al. 1991). Dietary diversity was positively related to nutritional status in an international sample of young children (6 to 23 months) (Arimond and Ruel 2004). Alternatively, dietary diversity within the sweets, snacks, condiments, entrees, and carbohydrate food groups is positively associated with obesity, while dietary diversity within the vegetable food group is negatively associated with energy intake and body fatness (McCrory, Fuss et al. 1999). Energy density is the major difference between diversity within foods positively associated with increased body fat versus the diversity of foods that are negatively associated (Clemens, Slawson et al. 1999). Consuming a wide variety of different types of non-nutrient-dense foods (chips, cookies, and candy) is associated with an increased BMI (Langsetmo, Poliquin et al. 2010).

Convenience

In today's society where both parents work in over half of married families, convenience is key when deciding what to eat. Fast food restaurants are an attractive option for families looking to find quick, low-cost meals. Unfortunately most fast foods are energy dense, contain lots of fat, have low fiber, and are available in huge portions (Bowman, Gortmaker et al. 2004), and regular consumption can lead to excess caloric intake, which may lead to weight gain. Children who consume fast food have a higher energy intake and lower dietary quality on that day than children who do not consume the fast food (Bowman, Gortmaker et al. 2004). In addition studies have shown that having fast food restaurants near schools increases the risk of the students being overweight (Davis and Carpenter 2009). Prentice and Jebb suggest in a review on fast foods and obesity that humans may not be able to compensate for the high energy foods by decreasing the amount they consume, thus leading to weight gain (Prentice and Jebb 2003). There will most likely always be fast food restaurants and millions of dollars spent on advertising fast food products to children and families. Advising families not to eat at fast food restaurants will likely not cause behavior change. Instead, educating families on how to make better choices when eating out or grabbing food on the go is most likely a more effective nutrition education strategy to use to promote positive behavior change.

Availability

Access to healthy foods can often be a barrier to eating a healthy diet in poor and rural areas in the middle of a food desert. A food desert is defined as an "area in the United States with limited access to affordable and nutritious food, particularly such an area composed of predominantly lower income neighborhoods and communities" (Ver Ploeg, Breneman et al.

2009). Many times these areas rely on convenience stores or fast food restaurants for food due to a lack of supermarkets or grocery stores. This can decrease access to fresh fruits and vegetables and lead to the purchases of foods high in added fats and sugars. Ease of access to supermarkets is another issue to consider. Rose et al. evaluated the relationship between ease of access to supermarkets and fruit and vegetable consumption in Supplemental Nutrition Assistance Program participants (Rose and Richards 2004). Seventy six percent of participants had relatively easy access to supermarkets based on distance and mode of transportation. Easy access was positively associated and distance to supermarket was negatively associated with fruit use. Ver Ploeg et al. expanded this study look specifically at fresh produce versus canned (Ver Ploeg, Breneman et al. 2009). Of the households evaluated, seven percent reported they did not shop mainly at a supermarket, which the authors attributed to limited access. This group purchased less produce and milk than frequent shoppers of supermarkets (at least once per week). Although the results of these studies indicate that lack of access or ease of access negatively affects the purchase of healthier food options, studies are needed to determine whether improving access would increase the purchase of these healthier foods.

Environment

According to Hill and Peters "one way in which the current environment promotes obesity is by providing more frequent opportunities for the consumption of large quantities of food (Hill and Peters 1998). A variety of highly palatable, inexpensive foods is available nearly everywhere." A cross-sectional survey of rural adults indicated that frequency of eating at establishments that promote excessive food consumption such as buffets, cafeterias and fast food was positively associated with obesity (Casey, Elliott et al. 2008). Young adults in the Coronary Artery Risk Development in Young Adults (CARDIA) study who ate at fast food restaurants more than twice a week had a significantly higher weight gain during the fifteen-year study period than those who ate there less than once a week

(Pereira, Kartashov et al. 2005). Despite these positive associations, a recent review of the literature indicates that there is not enough evidence to definitely support these associations and more studies are needed (Giskes, Kamphuis et al. 2007).

The marketing of energy dense, low nutrient foods is another environmental factor often recognized as contributing to the obesity problem in children and adolescents, with TV commercials representing 46% of all food marketing expenses to this age group in the United States. In 2006, this translated to over $745 million dollars (Harris, Schwartz et al. 2010). Eighty percent of all foods advertised during TV shows for children are for convenience/fast foods and sweets (Harrison and Marske 2005). According to Harrison and Marske a 2,000 calorie diet of foods advertised on TV would exceed sodium recommendations and provide one cup of added sugar (Harrison and Marske 2005). In addition to TV, food companies utilize radio, Internet, print media, and video games to influence kids with a total annual cost of approximately $10 billion a year (Medicine 2006). The Institute of Medicine published a report of a study they conducted to determine the influence food marketing had on children, and they concluded that advertising does influence what children eat as well as their health (Medicine 2006). This aggressive food marketing of less healthy food choices makes it difficult for parents to teach their children to eat healthier foods and undermines parents' authority (Center for Science in the Public Interest 2010). The Center for Science in the Public Interest has published guidelines for marketing to children designed to help food companies be more responsible (Center for Science in the Public Interest 2010). Adopting these guidelines is a great first step in supporting healthier dietary intakes in children.

Psychosocial Influences

There are many psychosocial factors that increase the risk for weight gain and obesity. Disinhibited eating, or disinhibition, was identified as a psychological construct associated with dietary control and attitudes toward food over twenty years ago (Stunkard and Messick 1985). Disinhibited eating is defined as "a tendency to overeat in the presence of palatable foods or other disinhibiting stimuli, such as emotional stress" (Savage, Hoffman et al. 2009). It has been positively associated with weight gain and BMI in a variety of studies (Savage, Hoffman et al. 2009; Hays, Bathalon et al. 2002; Lawson, Williamson et al. 1995; Williamson, Lawson et al. 1995). Bryant et al. recently published a review on the effect of disinhibition on appetite and weight (Bryant, King et al. 2008). They concluded that it is not only an important determinant of weight, but is also associated with less healthful food choices, eating disorders, low physical activity, and poor psychological health.

Certain emotional situations also can affect the amount of food consumed, which is referred to as emotional eating. People may use food as a coping mechanism to escape negative emotions experienced in certain situations (Bekker, van de Meerendonk et al. 2004). Weight status may influence the degree of food consumed during negative situations with overweight individuals reporting a higher food intake than their normal weight and underweight counterparts (Geliebter and Aversa 2003). Chronic depression has also been identified as a factor related to obesity, although it is not clear whether depression causes obesity or obesity causes depression. Recently, depression in childhood and adolescence has been found to be associated with a higher BMI in adulthood (Goodman and Whitaker 2002; Pine, Goldstein et al. 2001). Perhaps successfully managing depression in these age groups would decrease the risk of obesity later in life.

Stress also affects the way people eat, and there is a difference in eating patterns between responses to acute versus chronic stressors. Acute stressors invoke the "fight or flight" response, which tends to lead to a decrease in food consumption. More chronic stressors such as stress from a job, bad family situations, or financial hardships invoke a completely different hormonal pathway, which leads to elevated cortisol levels that appear to increase the desire to consume more tasty, energy-dense foods that can cause weight gain (Torres and Nowson 2007). Torres and Nowson reviewed human and animal studies on stress and weight gain and concluded that chronic stress may lead to overeating high energy foods that may in fact lead to weight gain, especially in men (Torres and Nowson 2007).

DIETARY STRATEGIES ASSOCIATED WITH A DECREASED OBESITY RISK

Factors associated with decreased obesity include some specific dietary intake patterns. "Nibbling" throughout the day (Summerbell, Moody et al. 1996) and consuming frequent meals (Metzner, Lamphiear et al. 1977; Fabry and Tepperman 1970;) are associated with lower adiposity. Eating breakfast (Summerbell, Moody et al. 1996; Schlundt, Hill et al. 1992) and consuming less energy during the evening (Summerbell, Moody et al. 1996) are also associated with decreased BMI. Increased consumption of meals outside of the home (Kant and Graubard 2004; McCrory, Fuss et al. 2000; McCrory, Fuss et al. 1999) and increased consumption of high energy density food (Kant and Graubard 2005) are associated with increased BMI.

Studies have also shown a link between obesity and skipping meals (Siega-Riz, Carson et al. 1998; Wolfe and Campbell 1993; Bellisle, Rolland-Cachera et al. 1988; Fabry 1970; Fabry and Tepperman 1970). Individuals who regularly consume breakfast have more adequate micronutrient intakes and better dietary quality than those who frequently skip breakfast (Nicklas, Myers et al. 1998; Siega-Riz, Carson et al. 1998; Sampson, Dixit et al. 1995). Eating a nutritious breakfast may help control body weight by reducing dietary fat intake and minimizing impulsive snacking (Ortega, Redondo et al. 1996; Schlundt, Hill et al. 1992). Although some people may believe they will reduce their caloric intake by skipping meals, an inverse relationship has been observed between frequency of eating and body weight, indicating that people who eat more often have a lower body weight (Summerbell, Moody et al. 1996; Kant, Schatzkin et al. 1995; Edelstein, Barrett-Connor et al. 1992; Dreon, Frey-Hewitt et al. 1988; Metzner, Lamphiear et al. 1977; Fabry, Hejda et al. 1966). Changes in food intake patterns may be contributing to overweight/obesity.

WHAT ABOUT PHYSICAL ACTIVITY?

The other side of the energy balance equation has to do with calories expended throughout the day. Again, if more calories are consumed than are burned then weight gain is the result. Americans have decreased their physical activity over the years. In addition to lack of time, which is a huge barrier to physical activity, there are other factors involved. This section will discuss these factors.

Built Environment

Throughout the obesity literature there is discussion on the impact that the built environment has on risk for obesity. The built environment encompasses a variety of things including but not limited to neighborhood walkability, access to parks, safety, cleanliness, and traffic flow (Renalds, Smith et al. 2010). These factors influence the ability and desire for people to be physically active. A review by Renalds et al. identified factors of the built environment that encouraged or discouraged physical activity (Renalds, Smith et al. 2010). More lights, less intersections and traffic, and better scenery all encouraged physical activity, while low security and poor neighborhood maintenance discouraged physical activity. Overall the authors concluded that neighborhoods that encouraged walking had more physical activity and lower incidence of overweight. Many studies have reported a positive association between some aspect of the built environment and obesity (Timperio, Jeffery et al. 2010; Papas, Alberg et al. 2007; Booth, Pinkston et al. 2005; Giles-Corti, Macintyre et al. 2003), possibly due to barriers to physical activity. Booth et al. state in their review on obesity and the built environment that biological, psychological, behavioral, and social factors do not fully account for the current obesity epidemic, which provides enough support to evaluate the effect of the built environment (Booth, Pinkston et al. 2005). Increasing the ability for neighborhoods to be physically active may translate into a reduced risk for obesity. This may be a challenge in socially disadvantaged neighborhoods where physical activity is lower for a variety of reasons (Turrell, Haynes et al. 2010; Cerin and

Leslie 2008; Giles-Corti and Donovan 2002). More affluent neighborhoods tend to have higher levels of physical activity, which may provide more protection against certain diseases in these communities (Turrell, Haynes et al. 2010).

Currently there are few published studies documenting the effect a change in the built environment has had on the community. McCreedy and Leslie describe a city-wide initiative in Orlando, Florida, called Get Active Orlando that brought together a multidisciplinary team of community partners passionate about changing the culture of their city to encourage physical activity (McCreedy and Leslie 2009). With a grant from the Robert Wood Johnson's Active Living by Design initiative, they were able to design and implement a community-wide campaign that encouraged healthy lifestyle changes. After establishing baseline data by surveying their target low socioeconomic status neighborhood, they developed programs designed to increase physical activity such as bike giveaways, safe bike rides, free bike repair, a senior walking program, and a community garden. These programs were successful in getting the community involved and physically active. The program successes have led to policy changes for development projects in the community intended to make the city more active. Their web site provides information as well as a Design Standards Checklist to be used by developers to promote physical activity in their developments. A similar program in Somerville, Massachusetts, (Burke, Chomitz et al. 2009) also achieved positive results. It is still too early to tell whether these changes will lead to a decrease in obesity in these communities, but they are definitely headed in the right direction. Other communities can look to Orlando and Somerville as examples of how a community can come together for the health benefit of their residents.

Screen Time

For years too much screen time, or time spent in front of any kind of screen, has been blamed for decreasing physical activity in children and adolescents. This includes television, movies, computer use, and video games. Current technological advances in gaming and the increased prevalence of movies and television targeted to children and adolescents has replaced the desire to play outside with friends or spend the weekends involved in organized sports in much of this population. According to a recent national survey, approximately 47 percent of children and adolescents two to fifteen years of age spend more than two hours a day in front of a screen (Sisson, Church et al. 2009). When separated by age the percentage of daily screen time greater than two hours a day was 33 percent, 6.7 percent and 47.3 percent in three to five, six to eleven, and twelve to fifteen year olds, respectively. The potential decrease in physical activity as a result of increased screen time may result in weight gain. Data from a cross-sectional study of children and television viewing in 1990 indicated that children who watched more than five hours a day of television were 4.6 times more likely to be overweight than those who watched zero to two hours of television per day. Parental weight status also seems to modulate the effect of screen time and BMI/body fat, with children of overweight/obese parents watching significantly more television and having higher BMI and body fat for every hour watched than children of normal-weight parents (Steffen, Dai et al. 2009). The American Academy of Pediatrics recognizes the potentially detrimental effect of too much screen time on children and adolescents, including negative behavior and obesity. Therefore, they recommend limiting screen time to less than two hours per day in children and adolescents and do not recommend any screen time for children under two years of age (Committee on Public 2001). There is provocative, new evidence that suggests that the obesity associated with television viewing in children may not be a result of a decrease in physical activity (Zimmerman and Bell 2010). Instead, television programming that includes commercials advertising unhealthy foods may be the factor. The authors recommend keeping children away from commercial advertising and directly encouraging physical activity as better strategies for addressing obesity than just limiting screen time (Zimmerman and Bell 2010). There is currently a lack of studies investigating the effect of screen time in adults. It seems to be more important to focus on lack of physical activity from a variety of factors.

Guidelines for Physical Activity

The Dietary Guidelines for Americans, 2005, include a set of specific physical activity goals to manage body weight and prevent gradual, unhealthy body weight gain or sustain weight loss. These guidelines specify the need for at least 60 minutes a day (60-90 minutes), on most days in a week, of moderate-intensity physical activity. Moderate-intensity physical activity is defined as any activity that burns 3.5 to 7 kcal/min resulting in reaching 60-73 percent of peak heart rate. Examples of moderate-intensity physical activity include brisk walking, bicycling, light yard work, and stretching.

Strength, flexibility, and cardiovascular exercise are three main categories of physical activity (Williams 2002). Considerations in physical activity include duration, intensity, frequency, and appropriate recovery time between activities (Williams 2002). Strength training activities are beneficial for improving body composition, body weight, and glycemic control (Sartorio, Maffiuletti et al. 2005; Dunstan, Daly et al. 2002;). Combining strength training and cardiovascular training may also improve insulin sensitivity (Ferrara, McCrone et al. 2004). Moderate, but not intense activity, is more effective at utilizing fat stores (Raguso, Coggan et al. 1995). Moderate level exertion leisure-time activities and common physical activities such as walking provide many health benefits (Laaksonen, Lindstrom et al. 2005; Littman, Kristal et al. 2005).

Summary

Obesity in America has increased significantly over the past forty years for a variety of reasons. The current obesogenic environment makes it easy to eat an excessive amount of calories without burning them. Understanding the barriers to proper nutrition and physical activity associated with an increase in risk for obesity is an important first step in the development of prevention and treatment programs.

Key Points

1. Obesity is at epidemic proportions in America.
2. Obesity is associated with eating too many calories and not getting enough physical activity.
3. At the same time many Americans are getting too many calories, they are not consuming enough of many essential vitamins and minerals.

Nutrition Practice Points

When counseling an individual, it is important to recognize and deal with your own internal judgments, preconceptions, and feelings about weight and obesity. As a health professional, you must enter into the education situation without bias and judgments. If you have repressed negative attitudes about weight, these attitudes may subconsciously affect the relationship you have with your client. Also, you need to recognize your client's complex emotional perspectives. Obesity is not a numbers equation for your clients; instead, it is a part of their lives that affects how they feel about themselves and how they are treated by the world. Whenever possible, obesity treatment should include a team of health professionals that includes a dietitian, a counselor, a certified personal trainer, and a doctor. Many patients will benefit from many other health professionals being involved in the management of their weight.

Terminology

Body Composition—The amount of muscle, fat, bone, and fluid in the body and their proportional amounts. It is what makes up the body.

Central Adiposity—Fat stored around the waist.

Dietary Diversity—Different types of food within the same food group. For example, dietary diversity would be eating many different types of vegetables from the vegetable food group.

Energy Density—The amount of calories provided per a gram of food. A vegetable would be a non-energy dense food because it does not provide many calories per gram of product. Peanut butter would be an example of an energy dense food.

Fat Utilization—The ability of the body to take fat that has been stored in adipose cells (fat cells) out of the cells to be used as energy.

Glycemic Control—The ability of the body to maintain blood glucose levels within physiologically normal values.

Glycogen—A storage form for glucose in cells that provides short-term energy.

HDL—High-density lipoproteins acts as the "garbage truck" for the body by taking cholesterol and triglycerides out of the blood and back to the liver to be reutilized or removed from the body. It is the "good cholesterol."

Insulin Response—After a meal is consumed, the body releases many hormones and chemicals to aid in digestion and absorption. Insulin is released from the pancreas to transport glucose in the blood to cells to be used as energy for cellular processes or to be converted into stored energy (as fat in adipose tissue) for use later as needed.

Insulin Sensitivity—The body's ability to use insulin to take up glucose effectively into cells to provide energy.

Isocaloric—Two different food items, meals, or dietary patterns that have the same amount of calories.

Lipolysis—The ability of the body to break down the fat that is stored in fat cells (adipocytes).

Nutrient Composition—The nutrients in a food item or meal.

Portion Size—The amount of food provided that is intended to be eaten at one time.

Quality of Life—Everything that influences a person's emotional well-being. Often this includes physical ability to take care of one's needs (dressing, feeding, cleaning), level of physical discomfort or pain, and physical ability to do what a person wants to do.

Socio-Economic Status (SES)—A person's social and economic status. SES often refers to many subjective factors including living environment, neighborhood environment, quality of housing, education, education level of close family members, and access to other economic related factors (clothing, cars, technology etc.).

Triglycerides—A glycerol backbone with three fatty acids attached. Most fats consumed in the diet are converted to triglycerides in the body. Having high levels of triglycerides in the blood is associated with having an increased risk of cardiovascular disease.

Visceral Fat (or Visceral Adipose Tissue Stores)—The fat found inside the body in between organs. It is different from subcutaneous fat found closer to the skin.

ACTIVITY

Find/take an image/photo and describe how the image/photo is related to food and weight.

Chapter 3

Environmental Influences on Food Behavior

Angela Bermúdez-Millán
and Rafael Pérez-Escamilla

Goal: This chapter examines aspects of the environment that influence food behavior.

Objectives: After completing this chapter, you should be able to:

1. Recognize aspects of your environment that influence your food behavior.
2. Identify disparities between differing communities' environments that may be related to differences in food behavior.
3. Describe methods that can be utilized in the environment to promote health.

Many factors in our environment affect our food behavior. It is important to understand these factors in a broader perspective, as part of a socio-ecological model (SEM). SEM is a useful model that helps understand the multilevel effects and interrelatedness of the macro (e.g. food price policies, social marketing), meso (neighborhood's social capital including access to healthy foods and opportunities for physical activity) and micro environments (e.g. household structure) and how they affect and interact with family and individual food choices and other lifestyle behaviors

(Fitzgerald and Spaccarotella 2009). SEM also helps explain how for example national, state and local food assistance policies and community outreach efforts can affect access to healthy foods at the neighborhood and household level. Indeed, heavy marketing by the food industry and economic factors that make unhealthy food (usually available in large portion sizes) appealing, inexpensive, highly accessible, and convenient are among the factors promoting an upward spiral in weight gain (Godfrey 2008).

In this chapter, we will focus on the influence of food marketing and the built environment, on food availability and access, as well as food behavior. These factors have all changed rapidly in the past one hundred years, and may be associated with the increase in obesity discussed in the previous chapter.

FOOD AVAILABILITY

More food is available today than ever before. Food is everywhere. When you think about what you will eat tonight for dinner, consider your many options. You could go to a restaurant, stop by a fast food place, microwave a prepackaged meal, or eat countless types and varieties of foods available in a grocery store. There are relatively few foods that you would not have access to if you had the money. One hundred years ago, when average people thought about what they would have for dinner, how many options did they have? Their options were very limited and would have depended on what could be grown locally, what the growing season had been like, and what they could prepare with very basic kitchen equipment. Do not forget how much time and work even a very simple meal requires when it is prepared entirely from scratch, with only home grown, harvested or hunted, and processed ingredients. Most people in America today do not have to consider those factors when deciding what to eat for dinner.

Many people have easily prepared, or already prepared, delicious foods available in the house when they wake up. On an average trip to work, a person may pass many fast food and quick service restaurants. To make food even more accessible, most of those fast food restaurants have a drive-thru so people do not have to get out of their cars. People at work are often exposed to foods they see and smell. Kind coworkers bring in treats to share and have candy dishes on their desks, making food even more available. Many worksites also have vending machines stocked with low-cost, high-calorie treats. Some offices have break rooms with fully functional kitchen areas. Many people have mini refrigerators in their office for convenient and quick access to food. For those who do not pack their own lunch, or have the option of being at home for lunch, there are plenty of restaurants near most worksites that provide a variety of options for lunch. In many urban areas, foods are also available from street vendors. Dinner options include grocery stores, home cooked meals, quick service restaurants, fast food restaurants, and convenience stores. When becoming conscious of food stimuli in the environment, it almost becomes easier to count the number of times there is no food present rather than to count the number of times food is present.

When we see food, see people eating, see pictures of food, or smell food, it acts as a prompt (conscious or unconscious) for eating. When we consider how many more prompts there are to eat in the food environment today as compared to one hundred years ago, it is hardly a surprise that many Americans are eating more than they need.

To restrict food intake to healthy levels in this food saturated environment, it takes constant conscious self-denial and control to make daily healthy intake decisions.

SCHOOL ENVIRONMENT

Some changes in the food environment have taken place relatively recently. The types of foods available in public schools have undergone recent transitions. In the 1980s and 1990s, many public schools began serving foods to keep their customers happy. The problem was that the customers were children or adolescents who knew very little about nutrition and cared even less about long-term chronic disease prevention. Hamburgers, French fries, pizza, and chicken nuggets became staples in many school cafeterias. Vending machines began providing sodas and other non-nutrient-dense snacks during and after school hours. In these emerging consumer driven cafeteria environments, many public schools began housing mini fast food restaurants. Many high school students began seeing Pizza Hut, Taco Bell, and other fast food companies sell their products in the public school cafeteria.

Many companies, such as Coke or Pepsi, were major financial supporters of schools and school affiliated sporting events. In exchange for the financial contributions, the food and beverage companies were allowed to advertise their products in the school environment. This financial relationship was very important to under-supported, financially disadvantaged schools. The food and beverage industry understood the value of establishing lifetime food habits and emotional associations with specific products that early introduction and repeated exposure creates.

At the same time that many negative dietary changes were occurring in the food environment, many schools were also reducing or eliminating opportunities for physical activity. Having unhealthy foods more readily available and allowing less opportunity for physical activity may also be related to the increases in childhood obesity rates that occurred in the 1980s, 1990s, and continued into the 2000s.

Recently, many schools have made voluntary or regulated changes to remove non-nutrient-dense foods from the school environment. Different school systems have developed different procedures and policies for sponsorship advertisements, vending machines, and *a la carte* cafeteria items. In addition federally funded programs such as the Supplemental Nutrition Assistance Program-education component (SNAP-ed) are now providing substantial funding for improving food and nutrition education in schools through innovative culturally and age-appropriate approaches including puppet shows (Perez-Escamilla et al. 2002). Many researchers are already seeing positive changes in dietary quality, weight, and behavior outcomes because of these policy changes that address the school food environment as well as the quality of nutrition education offered to the students.

HOME ENVIRONMENTS

The kinds of foods available in the home environment also affect food behavior. If healthy nutrient-dense foods are readily available in the home environment, adults and children alike are more likely to consume them. If non-nutrient-dense foods are available in the home environment, they are also more likely to be consumed. Simply providing visual cues (seeing them) for nutrient-dense foods will increase the consumption of those foods. If you walk by and see fresh fruit on the counter, you are more likely to snack on the fruit. When the fruit or vegetables are buried in the refrigerator, they are less likely to be consumed. A package of cookies is also likely to be consumed faster if left sitting on the table than if it is stored out of sight in the pantry. Upbringing and family influence can also impact food behavior. Fruit and vegetable consumption is a good example. A qualitative research study conducted among a diverse multi-ethnic population (Hispanics, African-American and Caucasians) documented that the early home food environment was perceived as affecting fruit and vegetable consumption later in life (Yeh et al. 2008). Hispanic participants reported the lack of familiarity with several fruit and vegetables available in this country and not knowing how to include them as part of their traditional dishes, limiting their consumption in the household.

BUILT ENVIRONMENT

Although the built environment includes many other features beyond food related establishments, food availability is largely a function of the built environment. The built environment is everything that physically is in the environment. This includes sidewalks, buildings, lighting, businesses, roads, cars, or anything else that can be physically seen or used.

The built environment influences food availability in many ways. In large urban areas, there is a growing problem of fewer grocery stores being available. When the financial value of space exceeds possible grocery store profits, other more profitable businesses take the place of those grocery stores. Another issue related to grocery stores and the built environment is transportation. In many large urban areas, some people do not have cars. People in urban areas often rely on public transportation. When a mother of three has to carry her groceries home on a bus, it will affect what type and how much food she purchases. Convenience stores, which may be more accessible to low income people living in urban environments than grocery stores, are less likely to have fresh fruits, vegetables and other nutrient-dense food options available. Additionally, the fruits and vegetables and other nutrient-dense food options that are available, tend to be of a lower quality and have a higher price. Research has shown that individuals living in lower socio-economic neighborhoods or higher minority population neighborhoods tend to have fewer grocery stores and more liquor stores. The accessible grocery stores in these areas have lower-quality/higher cost foods available, and clients may be subject to additional lending fees from store owners. For example, some local Hispanic convenience stores, also known as bodegas, allow clients from their communities to purchase foods under credit, a practice known in Spanish as *"fiado."* If a client needs a bag of rice, and/or a can of beans but does not have the money, she can go to the bodega and purchase these food items *"fiados."* The store owner then adds the debt to the client's credit file ensuring that the balance gets paid when the client receives food stamps or receives a pay check from work. Under the "fiado" system, some bodega owners, add an additional 'credit fee' to the already overpriced items. As a result, clients end up paying more money for their groceries, having less money to spend on food and other necessities for the next month, with the "fiado" cycle repeating itself increasing household food insecurity. Thus, policies that make it easier for bodegas to offer healthy foods at a reasonable cost (e.g., tax incentives), and that increase the purchasing power of their clients (e.g. increase in minimum wage) are likely to improve the food and nutrition security of the households in Hispanic inner-city neighborhoods. People living in rural areas may experience a similar lack of access to grocery stores. There are often fewer grocery stores, and the available grocery stores are often located very far from homes. In economically challenging and food insecure times, the additional cost for gas or the expense in transportation to a grocery store an hour or more away, is a hardship for many low-income families. Often times, individuals eat foods that are available to them in proximity to their homes. Accessibility to fast food restaurants is usually higher in low-income and minority neighborhoods, representing another neighborhood-level barrier for healthy eating (Block 2004).

The built environment also influences physical activity in many ways. If physical activity resources and facilities are lacking in the environment, people are going to be less likely to engage in physical activity. Lower socio-economic neighborhoods are less likely to have physical activity resources and facilities in their community. They are also more likely to have a built environment that has poor lighting, a lack of sidewalks, high traffic areas, an increased frequency of crossing streets, dogs off leashes, and higher rates of violent crimes than neighborhoods in more affluent areas.

You can see how the influence of the built environment on food availability and physical activity is hard to discuss without discussing the influence of economics. More on food availability and the built environment will be discussed in the economic influence on food behavior chapter.

MARKETING

Marketing is another significant part of the environment influencing food behavior. Historically, television advertisements have been considered the dominant marketing strategy for food/beverage products. Although television is still considered the most common strategy used, many other emerging and commonly used marketing strategies include: nutrition information on food labels, embedded marketing (e.g., product placement in television shows, movies, games, magazines, etc.), viral marketing ("word of mouth"), sales promotions (e.g., coupons, direct mailings, catalogs, etc.), co-branding (two different companies create one new product), cross-promotions (new products introduced and sold with existing products), marketing tie-ins (e.g., restaurants using movie promotional materials), premiums (e.g., toys or giveaways with product purchase), on-line promotions (e.g., games, targeted e-mailing, etc.), event and location marketing (e.g., school, sporting events, etc.), and wireless marketing (e.g., cell phones,

PDAs, pagers, etc.) (McGinnis 2006). Marketing campaigns may use many of these strategies in combination.

Nutrition Marketing on Food Labels

Although most nutrition and marketing research is focused on the impact of television advertising, nutrition marketing used on food labels and in food service may influence consumption patterns. Most consumers believe that food can help prevent disease and enhance health (Gilbert 2000). Product consumption is driven not only by product avoidance strategies, but also by health-promoting product seeking (Gilbert 2000). Health claims can alter consumers' perceptions toward specific food products (Bech-Larsen and Grunert 2003). Research has shown that products with health information on the labels influence consumer knowledge and behavior as well as company profits (Freimuth, Hammond et al. 1988). An example of increased profits from nutrition marketing is Eggland's Best nutritionally enhanced egg product. Eggland's Best experienced record sales growth after the introduction of their nutritionally marketed product (Michella and Slaugh 2000).

Increased consumer use of labeling information is related to having a higher quality of diet (Kreuter, Brennan et al. 1997). Most consumers use food labels. Consumers with higher levels of healthy eating behavior, self-efficacy, beliefs in diet-disease linkage and weight loss goals are more likely to use labels (Satia, Galanko et al. 2005). However, the majority of consumers cannot correctly interpret the labeling information (Fullmer, Geiger et al. 1991; Reid and Hendricks 1994; Levy, Patterson et al. 2000; Pelletier, Chang et al. 2004; Cowburn and Stockley 2005).

Labeling on packages may include nutrition facts, health claims, or nutrient content claims. The Food and Drug Administration (FDA) regulates the labeling of packaged processed foods. Only 1.7 percent of packaged processed foods are exempt from labeling requirements. The FDA allows health claims for foods that have sufficient scientific agreement linking the food to disease prevention (Rowlands and Hoadley 2006). They also allow "nutrient content" claims such as "100 percent Vitamin C" or "good source of protein."

Nutrient content claims are allowed without evidenced based research supporting a link of the nutrient to disease prevention (Katan and de Roos 2003). In 1997, only 4 percent of packages contained health claims and 39 percent of packages contained "nutrient content" claims (Brecher, Bender et al. 2000). In 2000-2001, 4.4 percent of food packages contained health claims and 49.7 percent of product labels had "nutrient content" claims (Legault, Brandt et al. 2004). Although research has not been conducted to determine how consumers differentiate between health claims and "nutrient content" claims, and how these claims impact food purchasing behavior, research in the tobacco industry has shown that consumers interpret allowed labeling claims of "No Additives" to imply that the cigarettes are healthier, less likely to harm and to be less addictive (Arnett 1999). Consumers may make similar extrapolations for products that contain "nutrient content" claims.

Price

Price is a tool in the marketing mix that may also be related to nutrition marketing practices (in addition to product, promotion, and place) (Kotler 1997). Price reductions in nutrient dense choices (low fat milk) in vending machines and cafeterias (fruit and vegetables) in the school environment positively influence sales (French, Jeffery et al. 2001; French 2003). Price may also be a barrier to healthy eating. Nutrient-dense foods are more expensive than non-nutrient-dense foods (Drewnowski, Darmon et al. 2004; Drewnowski and Darmon 2005; Andrieu, Darmon et al. 2006). Foods, such as margarine, with nutrition marketing (and less saturated and trans fats) have been found to be more expensive (Ricciuto, Ip et al. 2005).

Environment

Environmental changes in the marketing of food products can positively influence nutrient dense food purchasing behavior (Fiske and Cullen 2004). Having more nutrient dense foods available in a grocery store environment has been related to a higher diet quality of shoppers (Cheadle, Psaty et al. 1993).

However, increased nutrient dense food options in a restaurant environment does not necessarily equate increased sales; 46 percent of research and development directors of restaurant companies report that nutritious meal options represented 0-10 percent of sales (Sneed and Burkhalter 1991). Additionally, taste, quality, and appearance are more influential in meal selection than the marketing of health attributes of an entrée (Sproul, Canter et al. 2003).

One difference between foods in grocery store and in restaurant environments is point-of-purchase nutrition labeling. Most restaurants do not have point-of-purchase nutrition labeling, or if information is available, it has to be requested (O'Dougherty, Harnack et al. 2006). Most consumers surveyed supported laws that would require restaurants to include nutrition information on the menus (O'Dougherty, Harnack et al. 2006). The potential impact of menu nutrition information on consumer decision is currently being investigated (O'Dougherty, Harnack et al. 2006).

Social Marketing and Nutrition Marketing

Social marketing uses the tools from the commercial marketing sector in order to promote positive health behavior. Many positive changes have resulted from social marketing campaigns, including increased childhood immunizations, increased use of seat belts and bike helmets, smoking cessation (Brookes 2000), and breast feeding (McDivitt 1993). Social marketing has also been found to be effective in changing nutrition behavior (Braus 1995). In recent years there have been strong efforts at reaching out to minority communities living in the United States through culturally appropriate food and nutrition social marketing campaigns in diverse topics including breastfeeding (Stopka et al. 2002), fruit and vegetables (Pérez-Escamilla 2000), and food safety at home (Dharod et al. 2004).

Social marketing as a tool for behavior change is based in the Theory of Planned Behavior and Social Ecology Model (SEM) (Baranowski 2003). The Theory of Planned Behavior indicates that a person's behavior is influenced by attitudes, social norms, and perceived control over the behavior in question (Glanz 2002). SEMs of health behavior indicate that a person's behavior is influenced by institutional, cultural, and individual factors (Glanz 2002). The SEM has also been suggested to be the theoretical framework for SNAP social marketing efforts to improve diet quality, management of food resources, food safety, and food security (Gregson 2001).

The Theory of Reasoned Action is the basis of the Theory of Planned Behavior. The Theory of Reasoned Action can be considered when targeting a population with nutrition marketing seeking to improve specific health behavior (Booth-Butterfield 2004). This approach has been successfully applied in research settings such as a milk mass media campaign promoting "1 percent or less" as a nutrition intervention. The intervention utilizing nutrition marketing successfully altered attitudes, beliefs, and purchase intention (Booth-Butterfield 2004; Reger 1998). Changes in the availability of lower fat milk products in the bodegas or small convenience stores in the target community helped their nutrition marketing efforts to be successful.

Nutrition marketing with the goal of improving public health can be considered a form of social marketing. There are many examples of successful nutrition (social) marketing campaigns. One such example was the promotion of eggs and dark green leafy vegetables in Indonesia in order to reduce the incidence of vitamin A deficiency (de Pee 1998). In another example the "2 Fruit'n' 5 Veg Every Day" campaign in the Australian state of Victoria used television advertising to increase awareness, change beliefs, and increase consumption of fruits and vegetables (Dixon 1998). Similarly, the California Department of Health Services conducted a "5 a Day-for Better Health!" campaign, which successfully utilized mass media, the supermarket industry, and agribusinesses to increase awareness of health benefits and consumption of fruits and vegetables (Foerster 1995). A social marketing campaign in Bolivia, which used primarily radio and television advertising, was effective in increasing awareness and use of multivitamins (Warnick 2004). The "VERB" campaign, which used mass media, internet activities, and school and community program activities to promote daily physical activity, was successful in increasing awareness and activity (Huhman 2005).

Possibly one of the largest and most successful social nutrition marketing campaigns was conducted in New Zealand. The National Heart Foundation of New Zealand developed a symbol (a check mark called a "tick") for food labels indicating products meeting specific nutrient criteria. The "Pick the Tick" campaign resulted in many food companies reformulating their food products to meet the requirements to be eligible to display the symbol on the label and 59 percent of shoppers reported using the symbol to make food-purchasing selections (Young 2002).

NUTRIENT DENSITY SYMBOLS IN FOOD PRODUCTS

In the United States, the food industry, scientists and the United States Department of Agriculture (USDA) have developed 'nutrition quality' graphic symbols to help individuals make healthier food-purchasing selections. For example, when a food product meets the American Heart Association (AHA) certification criteria for healthy people over age two based on the saturated fat and cholesterol content of the product, it allows for a fee for the product to display its distinctive symbol of a heart and checkmark. This indicates to consumers that product is 'heart healthy' (AHA, Heart-Healthy Grocery Shopping Made Simple). The NuVal™ Nutritional Scoring System, attempts to summarize the overall nutritional value of a food product based on the Institute of Medicine's Dietary Reference Intakes and the Dietary Guidelines for Americans. NuVal™ takes into account the levels of more than thirty nutrients—including vitamins, minerals, fiber, and antioxidants; sugar, salt, trans fat, saturated fat, and cholesterol (Katz 2009). The system also incorporates measures for the quality of protein, fat, and carbohydrates, as well as calories and omega-3 fats based on scientific consensus. NuVal™ will be displayed right on shelf tags for purchase selection in supermarkets and grocery stores. As a response to the call from the 2005 Dietary Guidelines for Americans Committee to develop *"a scientifically valid definition of nutrient density to help with nutrition guidance,"* researchers in the United States proposed a new food nutrient

58

profiling system, a new model for ranking foods based on their nutrient composition, which could be used to help consumers improve their diets (Victor et al. 2009). Other efforts, such as front-of-package symbols (e.g. a traffic light: red, yellow and green), to better convey the nutrition characteristics of a food product are under consideration. The task has been very challenging as it is difficult to advise a consumer on a single food product selection without taking into account the overall dietary intake pattern of the individual. Also the implementation of these systems will require careful oversight to prevent misleading messages to consumers, as illustrated by the recent controversy of labeling a sugar coated breakfast cereal with the 'smart choice' symbol leading the FDA to push for an immediate halt to this program until it gets further reviewed (ABC News 2009).

MARKETING ON TELEVISION

Most research on the impact of marketing on behavior has been focused on marketing on television. Children are in an environment saturated with mass media primarily depicting negative behavior (Brown 2002). Children, on average, watch twenty-eight hours of television per week. This means, on average, children are exposed to 11,000 low-nutrition food advertisements per year. These low-nutrition advertisements have been found to result in an increase of total calorie intake (Jeffrey 1982). Eighty three percent of television food advertisements targeting children were found to be of convenience/fast foods and sweets primarily for snack time eating (vs. meals). Foods advertised would exceed the recommended daily values for sodium, total and saturated fat, and added sugars (Harrison and Marske 2005). Of 52.5 hours of Saturday morning children's programming, there were 997 commercials, 56.5 percent of which were for food. Forty-four percent of the food commercials were for foods classified in the fats, oils, and sweets section of the "Pre-MyPyramid" food guide pyramid (Kotz 1994). Similar research found that in the average 21.3 commercials children view in one hour, 47.8 percent of the commercials were food advertisements and of those 91 percent advertise food products high in salt, sugar, and/or fat (Taras 1995). Research in New Zealand found that food advertisements on children's television programming reflected a dietary pattern associated with the development of obesity and obesity related co-morbidities (cardiovascular disease, diabetes, and cancer) (Wilson 1999; Wilson 2005).

In addition to children, minority groups, such as African Americans, are targeted with marketing promoting fast food, soda, candy, and meats and less likely to be targeted with advertisements for grains, fruits, and vegetables than the general market advertisements. Of advertisements targeting African Americans, 14.9 percent made health claims (specific fat and weight) (Henderson 2005). Lewis and colleagues (2005) also identified substantially more advertising and promotion of unhealthful foods in restaurants in low-income African American communities in Los Angeles County (Lewis et al. 2005). Yancey and colleagues (2009) found out that the density of advertisements for high calorie, low nutrient-dense foods and beverages in four cities (Los Angeles, Austin, New York City and Philadelphia) varied by zip code area ethnicity, with African American zip code areas having the highest advertising densities, Latino zip code areas having slightly lower densities, and White zip code areas having the lowest. Researchers have also found when examining food commercials on television that of foods marketed as "low in cholesterol," 77 percent were high in fat and 43 percent of foods containing nutrition marketing were for non-nutrient dense foods such as artificial juice (Lank 1992).

Increased exposure to food advertisements is associated with increased food non-nutrient dense food consumption (Halford 2004). The more television children watch, the less fruit and vegetables they consume. It has been suggested this relationship is because of the increased intake of foods advertised on television replacing fruits and vegetables (Boynton-Jarrett 2003). Children in families with high levels of television usage obtain more of their calories from meat, pizza, sodas, salty snacks and less of their calories from fruit and vegetables than children in families with low levels of television usage (Coon 2001). Tanasescu et al. (2000) found in a Puerto Rican community in the United States a positive association between TV viewing and the risk of childhood overweight. An analysis of data on food advertising on television and prevalence of overweight individuals in the United States and eight countries in Europe and Australia, demonstrated a significant relationship between childhood overweight and frequency of advertisement of non-nutrient dense foods (Lobstein 2005).

Key Points

1. The environment is saturated with structural barriers that may influence food behavior. These include the built environment (including lack of access to healthy foods), and commercial marketing from the food industry.

2. Many of these environmental barriers disproportionately affect lower socio-economic strata, putting individuals of lower socio-economic status at increased risks for adopting unhealthy dietary and physical activity behavior, contributing to health inequities worldwide.

3. Marketing is an effective tool for changing behavior. Marketing can be used to promote unhealthy or healthy behavior. As proposed by Brownell and colleagues (Godfrey 2008; Schwartz and Brownell 2007) and fully supported by SEM, changing the environmental "default system" from facilitating access to unhealthy to healthy foods is key to turn around the obesity epidemic. Likewise, a better understanding of food cues (food quality, portion size, perceived healthfulness, and preparation time) as well as environmental cues (such as the presence of friends and family at the table, eating location, and the size and design of glasses and plates) is needed to change individual's food behavior in a sustainable way (Wansink et al. 2009; Wansink 2004).

Nutrition Practice Points

When working with clients, it is important to be aware of their environment and how it may influence their behavior. With this awareness, you can help the clients make choices and set goals for themselves that will address the barriers and negative influences posed by their environment. Strategies that you could suggest to your clients to help them make healthy food choices in an oversaturated food environment include:

- not shopping when they are hungry
- becoming consciously aware of advertisements that promote foods
- keep healthy snacks at work to help prevent snacking on less nutrient dense options available in the work environment
- keep healthy nutrient dense snacks in the car so they will not be tempted by restaurants in the environment they see as they drive home
- always shop at the grocery store with a list to help prevent impulse buys
- plan ahead for meals

Another approach health professionals can take to address and modify the influence of the environment on behavior is to support built environment planning. The emergence of urban "food deserts," areas within cities where low-income communities have poor access to fresh produce is a major problem (Beaulac et al. 2009; Smith and Morton 2009; Moore and Diez 2006). As health professionals, we can take an active role in writing grants and advising planning groups to mobilize or support the community's efforts to develop ideal built environments (community gardens, neighborhood grocery stores, neighborhood schools that children can walk to, sidewalks, adequate lighting, outdoor recreational facilities, neighborhood fitness centers, etc.). These built environment intervention strategies may have positive impacts on dietary quality and physical activity for the entire community.

Terminology

Co-branding—Two different companies working together to create one new product.

Cross-promotions—New products that are introduced and sold as a free sample or trial version with existing high selling products.

Embedded Marketing—Products that are placed in television shows, movies, games, magazines, etc. that are intended to affect the consumer on a subconscious level to create a craving for a product, establish emotions associated with a product, or develop a social norm associated with a product.

Event Marketing—Companies may pay to advertise their products at events (concerts, sporting competitions, conferences, etc) to increase awareness, interest and establish brand recognition.

Food Availability—All food available in the physical environment.

Health claims—The Food and Drug Administration allows health claims for foods that have sufficient scientific agreement linking the food to disease prevention.

Marketing Mix—Marketing professionals consider price, product, promotion, and place when designing a marketing campaign.

Marketing tie-ins—One company may use a new popular company, item, or event to promote their own products. An example of this would be a restaurant using movie promotional materials in their advertising. A new popular movie or event may draw attention to a company's advertisement that otherwise would have been overlooked.

Nutrient Content Claims— Marketing statements on food packages that list the nutrients in the product. Nutrient content claims are allowed without evidenced-based research supporting a link of the nutrient to disease prevention.

On-line promotions—Companies may use targeted emails to advertise products to customers. Some companies have on-line games available that help to create awareness, positive associations, and interest in their food products.

Premiums—Toys or other items that come with a product purchase. Premiums are intended to increase consumer interest and product sales.

Sales promotion—Products are marketed using coupons, direct mailings, and catalogs to create awareness and interest.

Social Ecological Model—These models of health behavior indicate that a person's behavior is influenced by macro, meso, and micro environmental factors and their interactions.

Social Marketing—The use of traditional marketing strategies to promote healthy behavior.

Theory of Planned Behavior—An extension of the Theory of Reasoned Action. It added the construct of perceived control to the theory.

Theory of Reasoned Action—This theory seeks to explain why people behave the way they do. The theory proposes that a person's behavioral intent (and thus behavior) is a result of their attitude toward the behavior and their perceptions of social norms associated with the behavior.

Wireless marketing—Companies may use wireless technology (cell phones, PDAs, pagers, etc.) to communicate information about their products.

Viral marketing—Messages about a product spread by "word of mouth." Viral marketing is used to increase interest and excitement in a product by getting people to talk about the product. Companies will sometimes pay a trendsetter to talk about the company's product with the trendsetter's friends and acquaintances or in a public setting.

ACTIVITY

For one entire day, keep track of all of your exposures to food. Include any time you see food (in person, on TV, in a movie, in an advertisement, on a billboard, etc.), smell food, or hear about food. How do you think these exposures influenced what you ate that day?

Chapter 4

Economic Influences on Food Behavior

Nicole Darmon and Pablo Monsivais

Goal: This chapter examines how economics influence food behaviors.

Objectives: After completing this chapter, you should be able to:

1. Understand monetary measures of foods and nutrients.
2. Describe the association between diet cost and diet quality.
3. Identify socioeconomic disparities in diet quality.
4. Recognize policies that can address economic barriers to nutritious food.

By some measures, the United States has the most affordable food supply in the world. In 2008, American households on average spent about 10 percent of their disposable incomes on food (Consumer Expenditure Anthology 2008). This wasn't always the case. In the 1890s, the proportion of income spent on food was 50 percent (Atkinson 1896) and in 1929, the proportion was nearly 25 percent. Since the 1930s, the proportion of income spent on food has steadily dropped, reaching the 10 percent mark for the first time in 1999. Economists have attributed this trend to rising incomes combined with changes to agriculture and food processing systems that have kept food prices down (Miller and Coble 2007).

With such an affordable food supply, why should we worry about economics when thinking about the many factors that influence food behavior? To put it simply, if food is "cheap," then isn't a healthful diet within reach of most everyone? In reality, economic factors are still a major driver of food choices and dietary patterns for most people (Glanz, Basil et al. 1998). The cost of food and other economic factors may be a major obstacle to a nutritious diet for many people. Studies have revealed substantial differences in food choices and diet quality among people of different socioeconomic status (Ricciuto and Tarasuk 2007). Moreover, people of lower socioeconomic status are disproportionately affected by obesity, diabetes, hypertension and other chronic diseases that are linked to diet (Drewnowski et al. 2007; Hayes et al. 2006).

The monetary cost of food affects food choices and dietary patterns. This chapter explores the economic dimensions of the food supply as well as how the cost of food relates to nutrition policies and public health. The goal is to provide an understanding of how the monetary cost of food affects what and how much we eat, and consequently the nutritional quality of our diets.

NUTRITION, HEALTH AND SOCIOECONOMIC STATUS IN INDUSTRIALIZED COUNTRIES

Although social inequalities in health cannot be summarized by inequalities in obesity, the social gradient in obesity has been the focus of much attention the last few years, no doubt due to the large "visibility" of the phenomenon, but also because of its paradoxical character, as poverty has been long associated with undernutrition rather than overnutrition. Indeed, throughout history, being poor meant being hungry. This is still largely true in much of the developing world. Today over one billion people worldwide are hungry or malnourished (FAO 2009). These people are often underweight and exhibit various signs of malnutrition due to the limited amount and variety of foods they are able to obtain. In contrast, the situation has changed in most industrialized countries, where the poor are more likely to be overweight or obese and suffer from diseases that are related to the excess consumption of calories and poor diet quality (FAO 2006).

The rise of overweight, obesity and chronic disease is one of the most significant and alarming public health trends in the United States and other industrialized countries. Between 1971 and 2006, the prevalence of overweight and obesity (BMI > 25) in U.S. adults rose from about 48 percent to over 73 percent (CDC 2008). Overweight and obesity increase the risk of diabetes, hypertension, cardiovascular disease and other chronic diseases (Popkin 2009). While these trends have affected most every segment of the population, some demographic and socioeconomic groups bear a disproportionate burden of obesity and chronic disease (U.S. Department of Health and Human Services 2000). Studies in the United States dating back to the 1960s show that the most disadvantaged groups suffer from higher rates of obesity. For both adults and children, the prevalence of obesity is inversely associated with socio-economic status, whether this is measured in terms of income or education level, or by the socio-professional category of the subjects (McLaren 2007; Sobal and Stunkard 1989).

A number of factors might explain this socio-economic gradient in obesity. Indeed, at every stage of life, the risk factors for obesity and overweight are more prevalent in poorer populations. At the beginning of life, babies born into poor families are likely to have an obese parent and/or have a mother who smoked during pregnancy, since the prevalence of obesity and smoking addiction are higher in these populations (Morbidity and Mortality Weekly Report 2008; Ogden et al. 2006). These babies also have an increased risk of being underweight at birth and are the least likely to be breast-fed (Wright et al. 2006; Dubois and Girard 2003; Li et al. 2002). All these factors are thought to increase the risk of future obesity (Proctor et al. 2003; Armstrong and Reilly 2002). Children and adolescents from disadvantaged environments are more sedentary (Proctor et al. 2003; Lee and Cubbin 2002), eat more often while watching television (Coon et al. 2001), eat less fruit and vegetables in terms of frequency (Haapalahti 2003), quantity (Xie et al. 2003; Neumark-Sztainer 2002) and variety (Kirby 1995), and consume more sugary drinks (Vereecken et al. 2005; Haapalahti et al. 2003; Serra-Majem et al. 2002; Laitinen et al. 1995) than children from affluent environments. These patterns typically persist into adulthood, so that low levels of physical activity and pronounced dietary imbalances give rise to overweight and obesity. Given these trends, the high prevalence of obesity among low SES populations is not surprising.

Diabetes and obesity are strongly linked to SES, and obesity is a major explanatory factor for inequalities in diabetes. All over Europe, countries with large disparities in obesity also have large inequalities in diabetes. In fact, there is much evidence that all diet-related diseases follow a socio-economic gradient (Mackenbach et al. 2008; Kunst et al. 1998). Indeed, inadequate food choices and sedentary lifestyles are the major causes of the worldwide obesity epidemics and increased risks of chronic disease including cardiovascular diseases, certain cancers and diabetes. Other diet-related disorders include dental caries (related to excessive and frequent intake of sugar and poor dental hygiene) and hypertension (related to excessive salt intake in susceptible population groups). Thus, health inequalities result in part from poor nutrition linked to socioeconomic disparities.

FOOD CONSUMPTION AND SOCIOECONOMIC STATUS

The kinds of foods individuals eat varies with age, gender, race and ethnicity and with their country of origin. Diets also differ among groups of different socioeconomic status. As early as the 1930s, scientists were documenting inadequacies in nutrition among people of lower socioeconomic status (Boyd-Orr et al. 1937). Socioeconomic status (SES) of an individual person or a household can be indicated by money income, educational attainment, occupation or a combination of these variables (Galobardes et al. 2007). Higher SES individuals are those with higher incomes and/or with higher levels of educational attainment and/or who have occupations that do not involve physical labor.

Typically, the diets of the low SES groups have a high energy density and a low nutritional value. Low SES groups are more likely to buy and to consume less vegetables and fruit, and in less variety. Other nutritious foods such as whole grains, lean meat, fish and shellfish are also consumed in lower amounts while refined grains and potatoes are eaten in larger amounts by low SES populations. These differences in diet composition translate to differences in nutrient intakes. Persons of higher SES consume more of the nutrients found in abundance in fruit and vegetables such as vitamin C, ß-carotene, potassium and folate (Darmon and Drewnowski 2008).

On the other hand the supplies of macronutrients, notably fats, do not differ substantially by the SES of the individuals (Darmon and Drewnowski 2008). This is because while adults of low socio-economic status consume higher quantities of added fats and fatty meat, they also eat more refined grain-based products and little cheese, so that they have a total fat intake not much higher than that observed in the general population.

High energy density and low nutrient density explain the high prevalence of obesity and nutritional deficiencies in the poorer groups (Shohaimi et al. 2004), notably in nutritionally vulnerable sub-groups such as the elderly (Berr et al. 1998), children (Schneider et al. 2005; Lehmann et al. 1992; Ford et al. 2002; Bates et al. 2002; Male et al 2001; Sherry et al. 2001; Spannaus-Martin et al. 1997), pregnant and breast-feeding women (Bodnar 2002; Duitsman et al. 1995), and people with known food insecurity, such as recipients of food aid (Kirkpatrick and Tarasuk 2008; Bhargava and Amialchuk 2007).

Barriers to Healthy Eating in Low SES Populations

Nutrition Knowledge

A number of factors have been cited to explain unhealthy eating habits in the low SES groups, including a lack of nutritional knowledge (Wardle et al. 2000), the rejection of preventive nutritional advice (Patterson et al. 2001), a lack of interest in long-term health (because short-term problems seem more important) and a mistaken perception of body weight (Jeffery et al. 1991). However, even though it is true that nutrition knowledge is more common among higher SES populations, that knowledge is not necessarily associated with SES, regardless of SES. (Dallongeville et al. 2001). Qualitative surveys of poor people underline the isolation at mealtimes and the lack of interest in cooking (Roux et al. 1999). Several studies suggest, nevertheless, that low income groups possessed adequate cooking skills (McLaughlin et al. 2003). In France, (Perrin et al. 2002) as in the United Kingdom (Caraher et al. 1998) and the USA (West et al. 1999), it is the middle classes who do the least cooking and make the most use of ready meals and takeaways.

Psychosocial Factors

Poverty is often accompanied by solitude, boredom and depression, leading to more time being spent in front of the television. This leads to a risk of weight gain, not only because watching TV is a sedentary activity, but also because the people who watch it often are more exposed to advertising for food of low nutritional quality and high energy content (Wilde 2009). Dietary choices are subject to pressure from advertising and marketing by the food industry, which is designed to influence consumer behavior. However, it has been shown that social networks and social support limits the risk of unhealthy eating, whereas social vulnerability (isolation and loss of self-esteem) increases it (Martin et al 2004; Mazur et al. 2003; Darmon and Khlat 2001).

This may explain some paradoxes observed in low SES populations, such as the lower rates of breast-feeding. Low-income mothers often have low self-esteem and are apt to regard their breast milk as inferior to commercially-prepared baby formula. This illusion is maintained by the relatively high price of these formulas, which are usually abandoned in favor of simple semi-skimmed cows' milk (Dubois and Girard 2003), with the associated risks of iron deficiency and future obesity (Bonuck et al. 2002; Rolland-Cachera et al. 1995). This psychological, social and economic vulnerability of the parents explains another frequently-quoted paradox, which is the purchase of national brand snack foods by poor families, even when less-costly alternatives are available. This allows the children to socialize and "fit in" with other children for little cost. Also, it is difficult to refuse one's children a treat when it is all one is able to offer them.

Physical or Geographical Factors

The eating habits of individuals can be shaped by the physical make-up of their neighborhoods. Studies conducted in the US and UK have shown that low-income or low-SES neighborhoods in urban areas often have access to fewer options when shopping for food. Such neighborhoods lack supermarkets or other larger grocers offering a variety of nutritious foods. So-called 'food deserts' have been reported in low-SES urban areas and also in rural areas (Beaulac et al. 2007).

Areas identified as food deserts usually have food stores, but these are often convenience stores or other small shops that have higher prices and less selection than supermarkets. Moreover, the nutritional quality of items in smaller shops is typically lower than what would be available in supermarkets. Consumer access to supermarkets appears to have beneficial effects on the diet quality. According to North American (Morland et al. 2007) and British (Cummins 2003) studies, the nutritional quality and dietary choices are better when the individuals have easy access to a supermarket.

Financial Access

For persons of low SES, food budgets are usually low in absolute terms but can make up a large part of the total budget. For instance in France, households belonging to the lowest income group spent less than 10 Euros per day for food at home, but this small amount represented nearly a quarter of the total budget of these households (**Figure 4.1** (Caillavet et al. 2006). Thus, the amount of money spent on food in fact decreases when the percentage of income spent on food increases. This trend reflects a basic economic principle first described in the 1850s by Ernst Engel. Engel's Law states that as income rises, the proportion of income spent on food falls, even if absolute expenditure on food rises. Therefore, poor people have to face a double economic constraint on food: first, they only have a low amount of money to spend on food; second, this little money weighs heavily on their total budget.

Figure 4.1. Absolute and relative expenditures on food in relation to household income, in France.

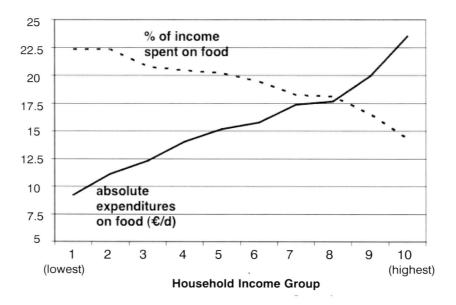

Adapted from Darmon M, Darmon N. (2008) L'équilibre nutritionnel. Concepts de base et nouveaux indicateurs: le SAIN et le LIM. Tec&Doc Lavoisier Editeur.

It is likely that this double constraint adversely affects food choices. In an analysis of Canadian food budget surveys, the strongest positive relation between income and the quantities of food purchased was found for fruit and vegetables (Ricciuto and Tarasuk 2007). This raises the question of whether economic constraints may drive people to make unhealthy food choices. Are healthy foods and healthy diets more expensive than unhealthy ones? This will be explored in the next sections of this chapter.

Monetary Cost of Food

Defining the Cost of Food:
Per Packet, Per Gram and Per Unit Energy

Food prices are something that most of us think about. We may read sale circulars, clip coupons or browse the Internet to guide us to the best 'deals' in groceries. We are accustomed to seeing prices for skim milk, bread and tomatoes expressed as "per half-gallon," "per loaf," and "per pound" respectively. Since shelf prices can reflect the cost of different units, it is essential that we standardize the calculation of food prices in some way to better understand how prices shape food choices and diet patterns.

One way is to transform shelf prices into prices per a fixed unit of weight. If we assume the example foods mentioned above have the same unit price of $1.99, then the milk prices of $1.99/half gallon would be transformed to $0.10/100 grams (**footnote 1**). Bread that was $1.99/loaf would be $0.39/100 grams (for an 18 oz loaf). Tomatoes at $1.99/pound would be $0.48/100 grams. Notice that this begins to allow direct comparisons of food prices among foods that are sold in different types of packaging and in different unit weights. This standardization will become even more important in discussions about the cost of food energy and nutrients, which will follow.

The Hierarchy of Food Prices:
Costly Calories, Cheap Calories

The different methods of measuring the cost of food reveal some important trends that have implications for nutrition and health. Measuring the cost of food per unit weight is one way to standardize the analysis of food prices. Another way is to standardize prices to the nutrients and calories contained in foods. The various foods and beverages available to consumers differ substantially in their nutrient composition. This was noted over one hundred years ago by the early nutrition scientist Wilber O. Atwater, who wrote:

"In comparing different food materials with respect to their cheapness or dearness, we are apt to judge them by the prices per pound, quart, or bushel without much regard to the amounts or kinds of actual nutrients which they contain. Of the different food materials which the market affords and which are palatable, nutritious and otherwise fit for nourishment, what ones are the most economical?"

Table 4.1. Standardizing cost of foods by weight, energy and nutrients

	$ / 100g	$ / 100 kcal	$ / 50 g protein	$ / 75mg vitamin C
Milk, skim[a]	0.10	0.27	1.39	37.50
Bread, wheat	0.39	0.15	1.79	29.25
Tomatoes, fresh, raw[b]	0.48	2.67	26.67	2.77

All prices based on a Seattle-area supermarket, October 2009. **a** For milk, $/100g based on 1,960 grams per half gallon. **b** For tomatoes, $/100g takes into account edible portion only. Nutrient data from the USDA's National Nutrient Database for Standard Reference 21.

Atwater (Atkinson 1896) recognized that consumers need to balance their monetary food budget—the amount of money they can spend on food with their nutritional requirements, the amounts of energy (kilocalories) and nutrients that are required to sustain health. In the US, nutritional requirements are embodied in the Dietary Guidelines for Americans, which make gender- and age-specific recommended intakes for energy and a range of macro- and micro-nutrients (*The Report of the Dietary Guidelines Advisory Committee on Dietary Guidelines for Americans 2005*).

To better understand how consumers may reconcile monetary budgets and nutritional goals, we must first express the cost of food in terms of nutrients and energy. In the milk, bread and tomato example described above, we noted that the same shelf price for the three items translates to different costs per 100 grams. Milk, bread and tomatoes do not contain the same energy or nutrient levels, so prices can be expressed to reflect these differences. **Table 4.1** shows how the relative prices for these three foods vary when price is expressed per 100g, per 100 kcal, and per ration of protein and vitamin C. While the cost of food standardized per 100g varies between 10 cents and 48 cents, the cost per 100 kcal varies more substantially. In this example, bread is the least costly source of calories while tomatoes are the most costly, in fact about 18 times more expensive. Similarly, the cost of obtaining a standard quantity of protein can vary even more. For these three foods, the cost of obtaining 50g of protein, is lowest for skim milk and highest for fresh tomatoes, which is not surprising given that tomatoes do not contain appreciable amounts of protein. When cost is standardized in terms of vitamin C however, the trend reverses, with tomatoes proving to be the lowest-cost source of this nutrient. Note that in this simple example of three food items, the most economical food was different when cost was standardized in terms of energy (bread), protein (milk) and vitamin C (tomatoes). Analyses of this type are important in helping consumers meet nutrition goals within a budget.

Whether or not healthy recommended foods are more expensive than others has been addressed by studying the relationship between the per-calorie cost of food and indicators of food nutritional quality, such as the Nutrient Density Score. Based on French data, **figure 4.2** shows that the meat and fish group, and the fruit and vegetables groups have the highest nutrient density but they also have the highest energy costs (Maillot 2007; Darmon 2005). In contrast, energy-dense foods such as sweets and salted snacks have the lowest nutrient density and they also are one of the least expensive sources of dietary energy. Dairy products occupy an intermediate place in this hierarchy. Starches and grains are interesting in terms of nutritional quality to price ratio because they are low in nutrients to be limited (sodium, fat, sugar) yet they provide energy at a low cost. Thus, with the noteworthy exception of starchy foods, it can be concluded that foods habitually recommended for a healthy diet, such as fruit and vegetables, lean meat and fish are often more expensive than energy dense foods, Results also showed that, within each major food group, some

Figure 4.2. Energy Cost and Nutrient Density Score of the Main Food Groups, Based on French Data.

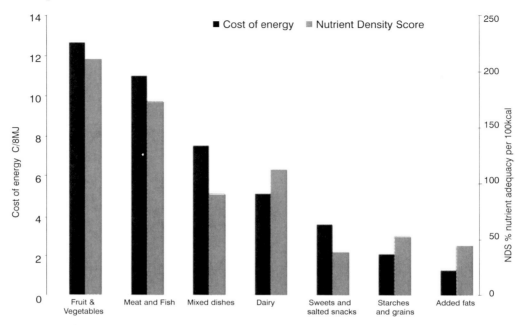

Data from reference (Maillot et al. 2007)

subgroups and some foods had a higher nutritional quality to price ratio than others, which explains how it is possible to construct nutritious foods at a moderate cost (Maillot et al. 2008). However, globally, the current structure of food prices does not seem to favor the consumption of diets that are low in energy density, rich in fruit and vegetables, and of high nutrient density.

Cost of a Healthy Diet

Is It More Expensive to Eat a Nutritious Diet?

Until recently, this is a question that has received little attention from researchers. Researchers or others who are concerned with identifying barriers to healthful eating have historically not considered food prices to be a major issue, at least in developed countries. Sociologists and anthropologists have shed light on this issue, by demonstrating that low SES individuals face many barriers to eat healthily (Dowler and Dobson 2007). Such studies also showed that perceived economic barriers have a main impact on food choices and patterns of eating in these populations. For example, low-income mothers reported that they know the basis of what constitutes a balanced diet, that they would like to eat fruit and vegetables more often and to give them to their children, but that they can't afford them (Dammann and Smith 2009). In addition, several reports describe low-income women as wise shoppers with adequate cooking skills, concerned with cost and quality (McLaughlin et al. 2003; West et al. 1999). Thus, a recent study showed that, when asked what foods they would add if they were given an additional 25 percent of their budget to spend on food, low-income women chose more foods from the 'healthier' categories, again highlighting the importance of cost when making food choices (Inglis et al. 2009). Clearly, these studies raise concerns about the potential increases in the financial cost of following a diet that complies with dietary guidelines.

Beyond consumer perceptions, the question of whether it is actually more costly to eat healthily has not been directly addressed until the last decade. Methodological considerations may partly explain this delay, since economists, who have very detailed information on household food expenditures typically lack data on individual food and nutrient intakes, while nutritionists, who have developed methods to precisely assess food intakes and nutritional adequacy of diets, generally lack information on the price paid by individuals for the food consumed. In the 1990s, the fields of consumer economics and nutrition began to converge, making it possible to either link food prices with dietary surveys or to link nutrition data to surveys on consumer expenditures (Bowman 1997; Huang 1996). Below, we review four major types of studies that have examined the cost of a nutritious diet.

Research Studies on the Cost of Nutritious Diets

Cross-Sectional Studies

Cross-sectional studies are observational and generally involve study of a sample of people at one point of time. As such, they provide a snapshot of conditions. An Australian study examined the cost of healthful eating using dietary data from the national dietary survey and data on food and drink prices collected in supermarkets and other food outlets (McAllister et al. 1994). This study found that diets of those persons who complied with dietary guidelines paid more per unit of energy (kcal) than those whose diets did not comply with guidelines. Moreover, in a diet modeling exercise, the researchers examined the effects of substituting nutritious foods into the typical Australian diet, which they had found to be of poor nutritional quality. While this substitution led to a modest improvement in the average Australian diet, it raised the total cost of the diet (McAllister et al. 1994).

Later studies generally made similar findings. In a diet and nutrition study of more than 15,000 women in the UK, researchers estimated the monetary cost of diets and correlated these cost estimates with a diet quality indicator based on dietary recommendations from the World Health Organization (Cade et al. 1999). The results showed that healthier diets were those that were also the most expensive, both per day and after adjusting for energy intakes. In addition, fruit and vegetable consumption were shown to be the main items making a healthy diet more expensive. This observation was not surprising given that fruits and vegetables are some of the most costly sources of dietary energy. Studies from France and Japan showed that energy dense diets cost less than energy-dilute diets (Darmon et al. 2004) and that the most costly diets were rich in fruit and vegetables and low in sugars, refined grains and fats (Drewnowski et al. 2004). Studies in Spain produced similar findings where diet quality was assessed on the basis of adherence to the Mediterranean diet pattern, which has been associated with positive health outcomes (Lopez et al. 2009; Schroder et al. 2006). More recent US-based studies have also shown that diet cost and diet quality are positively associated in low-SES populations (Townsend et al. 2009) and in higher-SES populations (Monsivais 2009).

At a first glance, it seemed that the positive relationship between diet quality and diet cost might be driven by the low cost of fat and sugar in foods and their high energy density (Drewnowski 2003). Indeed, energy dense foods were shown to be cheaper sources of energy than energy-dilute foods such as vegetables and fruits. Also, the fact that nutritious diets tend to be energy-dilute implies that eating a more nutritious diet requires consuming greater bulk, i.e., eating more (volume and/or grams of foods).

However, nutritious diets are not simply defined by their low energy density. Nutritious diets also have a high content of vitamins and minerals because they are rich in vegetable and fruits, whole grains, lean meats, fish, and other foods characterized by a high nutrient density (Schroder et al. 2008; Ledikwe et al. 2006). So is the higher cost of more nutritious diets due to the lower energy density or is it the case that nutrients in the diet are also costly? This question was addressed using data from a French national dietary survey. The researchers stratified adult participants by quartiles of dietary energy cost (in terms of Euros/10 MJ) and dietary energy density, total energy and nutrient intakes were then compared across groups (Andrieu et al. 2006). As shown in **Figure 4.3,** participants in the lowest level of energy cost had the highest energy intakes, the most energy dense diets and the lowest daily intakes of key vitamins and micronutrients. Participants in the highest level of energy cost had lower energy intakes, and their diets were higher in nutrients and lower in energy density (**See footnote 2**). The findings indicate that those in the highest group of dietary energy cost tended to chose foods with a high content of nutrients and moderate energy content, namely the nutrient dense foods, fruit and vegetables.

Figure 4.3. Daily intakes of energy and selected vitamins among four levels of energy cost of diets of adults living in France.

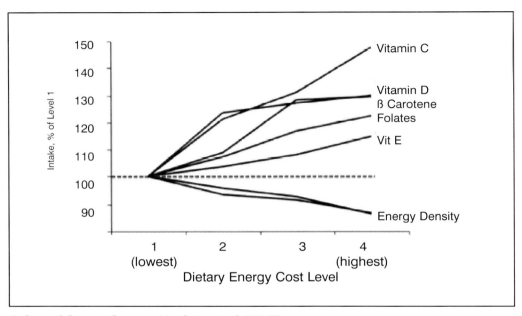

(adapted from reference (Andrieu et al. 2006))

A separate analysis of the same French data found that diets of higher nutrient content (calculated using the mean adequacy ratio -MAR- of diets, based on the intake of 23 essential nutrients) were associated with higher diet costs, and that this relationship was independent of the relationship between diet cost and energy density (Maillot 2007). For a given energy intake and energy density, each 10 percent increase in MAR led to a 13 percent increase in estimated diet costs per 10 MJ. From these findings, the researchers concluded that higher-quality diets cost more not only because they had a low energy density but also because they were nutrient rich. Accordingly, a recent Spanish study showed that higher energy cost was associated with higher likelihood of meeting nutrient-based recommendations (Lopez et al. 2009).

To date, cross-sectional studies indicate that nutritious diets carry a price premium. However, like all observational studies, the cross-sectional studies described here have a number of technical limitations related to their dependence on reported dietary intakes and retail food prices rather than actual expenditures. But the most significant limitation of observational studies is that their conclusions are based on correlations. They can't provide evidence for causality. In other words, cross-sectional studies can merely indicate a link between dietary quality and diet cost, but they do not address the question whether healthy diets are more costly because of their high dietary quality. Moreover, most of these studies did not control for SES variables. Thus, researchers could not exclude the fact that confounding factors, in particular the education status and/or the income level, may explain why individuals that have healthier diets also have diets that cost more. Interestingly, the US observational studies found the positive relationship between diet quality and cost to be true in both low-income populations (Townsend et al. 2009) and among higher income populations (Monsivais 2009). However, these results alone are not a direct demonstration of a causal relationship between diet quality and diet cost.

Longitudinal Studies

Other observational studies that might provide evidence as to whether nutritious diets are more costly come from longitudinal studies, in which each participant is studied initially then subsequently tracked over a defined period of time. Some longitudinal studies have shown that an involuntary decrease in household income (Köhler et al. 1997) or threats to employment security (Ferrie et al. 1998) each induced an increase in body weight. However, it was not known whether such weight gain was directly due to unfavourable changes in dietary patterns or to other behavioural changes, such as a decline in physical activity for instance. More recently, it has been shown among low-income food insecure individuals that the decrease of household resources at the end of the month was associated with a decrease in the quality of the diet, in particular the consumption of fruit and vegetables declines as resources become depleted (Tarasuk et al.

2007). This, again, strongly suggest that economic constraints have an unfavorable impact on diet quality. However, it is still not known whether their deleterious impact on food choices is direct, or indirect, by modifying psychosocial factors, stress and self-esteem in particular.

Intervention Studies

An alternative to observational studies is the intervention study. Intervention studies are experimental in nature and are designed to test the effects of some intervention or action (usually performed by the researcher) on some outcome of interest. In the field of nutrition, intervention studies to improve diet quality have generally examined the impact of nutrition education on a variety of outcomes. Studies on the effects of nutrition education on the quality and cost of the diet have led to conflicting results. Some found that interventions that improved the quality of the diet also increased the cost of the diet (Stender et al. 1993) while others either found no difference (Goulet et al. 2008; Mitchell et al.) or even a decrease (Ottelin et al. 2007; Burney and Haughton 2002) in food expenditures. Another study, conducted in 20 American families with at least one obese child, 20 weeks of an intervention aimed at increasing nutrient density did not change the cost per 100 kcal of diet, but decreased daily diet costs because of the decrease in energy intake induced by the intervention (Raynot et al. 2002). Likewise, in the two other studies that have reported a decrease in diet cost, it was acknowledged that such a decrease was in fact due to a decrease in energy intake, although this was not clearly specified. Interestingly, in a very recent study conducted in healthy women in Canada, a nutritional intervention promoting a Mediterranean pattern of eating neither increased daily diet costs nor did it increase the energy cost of diets, after 24 weeks of intervention (Goulet et al. 2008). Thus, although individuals who spontaneously adopt a Mediterranean dietary pattern were previously shown to have a more expensive diet than those who did not (Lopez et al. 2009; Schroder et al. 2006), individuals who were encouraged to adopt it did not increase their diet costs (Goulet et al. 2008). In accordance with the conclusion of McAllister (McAllister et al. 1994), this suggested that a healthy diet need not to be more expensive than a less healthy one.

Diet Simulation

Even intervention studies have not been able to clearly answer the causality question, not only because they were not double-blind studies, but more importantly, because they were not aimed at modifying total income or the budget for food. Indeed, the gold standard way of addressing causality in epidemiology is to undertake controlled double-blind randomized interventions. In our case, the intervention would consist of experimentally increasing or decreasing the budget for food in order to observe the possible changes in dietary quality induced by this intervention. However, such interventions are not feasible for a number of reasons. A more realistic approach to exploring cause and effect is through diet simulation studies.

Diet simulation allows researchers to explore how consumers' diets might vary depending on a range of conditions. The simulations are run on a computer and rely on mathematical models that can be programmed with a variety of constraints including nutrient goals, food composition and the total monetary cost of the simulated diet. An obvious advantage of diet simulation is that researchers can use the technique to study in isolation the impact of a cost constraint on food selection and related nutritional quality. Moreover, researchers can impose constraints on the computer's "diet" that would not be ethical (or even possible) to impose on the diets of real people. For example, the cost of the simulated diet can be reduced in order to test whether reducing diet cost necessarily results in a reduction in its nutritional quality. The results showed that the computer model was able to decrease diet cost by decreasing fruit, vegetables, meat and fish intakes and increasing the intake of refined grains (Darmon et al. 2002). The result was lower nutrient content and higher energy density of the cost-constrained simulated diet (Darmon et al. 2003; Darmon et al. 2002). These results are striking partly because they resembled the food intake patterns observed among low socio-economic groups. Making the cost constraint more severe induced such a deterioration of diet quality, that it could be viewed as a caricature of what would happen if we were only guided by economic considerations when making food choices.

With the knowledge that economic constraints can have a strong and unfavorable impact on food patterns and diet quality, an important question to address is whether nutrition education might attenuate the negative impact of economic constraints on diet quality. Again, diet simulation approaches provide an excellent tool to answer this question. Indeed, models can be designed, in which a food budget constraint simulates economic constraints, while constraints on nutrients (i.e. constraints based on nutritional recommendations) simulates nutrition knowledge and the willingness to eat healthily. In addition, constraints on foods and food groups can be included to guarantee that the modelled diets globally follow the same patterns as those observed in the general population, therefore ensuring them a certain level of social acceptability. Applied to both French (Maillot et al. 2010) and US data (Wilde and Liobrera 2009), such models showed that nutritional and social acceptability constraints both increase diet costs. Indeed the minimal cost of simulated diets increased with increasing level of nutritional standards and with increasing stringency of social acceptability constraints. In other words, forcing the simulated diet to be more nutritious and/or more in line with social norms of food consumption resulted in a higher diet cost.

Time Requirements of a Healthy Diet

Along with cooking skills, money and other resources, time is one of the resources necessary for the production of nutritious meals. People are spending less time preparing and eating food, which might have consequences for nutrition and health. Studies of time use show that between 1965 and 1998, the amount of time Americans spend in food preparation fell by nearly 40 percent to 27 minutes per day (Jabs and Devine 2006). Fresh produce, whole grains, beans and lean meats and seafoods—in other words the most recommended foods from the standpoint of nutrition—can be time and labor intensive to prepare. Studies have found that the time required to prepare low-cost, nutritious meals was greater than what most households dedicate to food preparation (Rose 2007; Davis and You 2006). When less time is devoted to food preparation, consumers often turn to processed or other ready-made foods that might be more energy dense and contain fewer nutrients (Drewnowski and Darmon 2005). There are few studies on the time cost of a nutritious diet but it is clear that when faced with limited time, consumers are likely to turn to restaurant meals, and in particular, fast foods, which are palatable and convenient (Stewart et al. 2006).

Public Policy Answers to Improve Nutrition in Vulnerable Groups

Public policies can be used to address poor nutrition in the general population and reduce disparities in diet quality. Public policies are generally based on the notion that poor nutrition is either due to poverty and lack of resources and/or lack of nutrition knowledge. Public policies include the programs, laws and regulations that can provide resources and information for the purchase of nutritious foods. Public policies can also influence the price of foods through subsidies and taxes. Below we review a variety of public policies at the federal, state and local levels that have the potential to improve consumer access to nutritious food.

Food Assistance Programs

Food assistance programs provide direct support to low-income individuals and families for the purchase of food. In the US, a variety of nutrition programs are administered by the USDA, each operating through different channels. For pregnant women and families with small children, the Special Supplemental Nutrition Program for Women, Infants and Children or "WIC" program provides vouchers for specific foods that are rich in nutrients needed for this sub-population. Alternatively, the Supplemental Nutrition Assistance Program (SNAP), commonly known as the "food stamp program," provides monetary benefits that are redeemable on most all foods but not alcoholic beverages or tobacco. Children in participating childcare homes or programs benefit from the Child and Adult

Care Feeding Program, which provides payments for food that meets particular nutritional criteria. For children in public schools, USDA's School Breakfast and National School Lunch Programs provides free or reduced meals that meet federal standards for nutrition.

For the WIC, the SNAP and the school meal programs, eligibility is based on household income and the number of people in the household. From this information, households are deemed eligible if household income falls below specific thresholds used in defining poverty.

Participation in these programs is intended to promote food security, which is the access to enough nutritious food for an active, healthy life. High rates of obesity in the poorest segment of the population, including those families on food assistance, has prompted controversy over the possible role of these programs in promoting obesity. Research on the impact of these programs on nutrition and health have shown varied results. WIC participation has been shown to promote the growth and health of infants and children while not contributing to childhood obesity (Ver Ploeg 2009; Black et al. 2004). Several studies have shown that SNAP participants have higher BMIs on average than similar people who do not participate (Zagorsky and Smith 2009) and some researchers have suggested that the program promotes the overconsumption of food in general and energy-dense, nutrient-poor food in particular. However, the available data are not sufficient to clearly place any blame on program participation itself.

More recent food aid programs have tried to promote the consumption of nutrient dense, energy dilute food directly. Pilot programs in the US and UK have tested the effect of increasing the economic yield of food stamps when they are used to buy fresh produce. This strategy effectively narrows the disparity in cost/kcal of nutrient dense foods and energy dense but nutrient poor foods. Studies on the programs indicate that providing vouchers for purchasing fruit and vegetables was a simple and effective way of increasing fruit and vegetables intakes among low-income women, while dietary advice alone had no great effect (Herman et al. 2008; Burr et al. 2007).

Be they conducted in the UK (Nelson et al. 2002; Morris et al. 2000), in France (Darmon et al. 2006), in the US (Cassady et al. 2007) or in Canada

(Vozoris et al. 2002), virtually all the studies that have estimated the minimum food budget needed to eat healthily have concluded that people living under the poverty level do not have enough money to spend on food, or that the dietary changes needed to meet the guidelines at an affordable cost are not likely to be acceptable, be it on a social or on a behavioural point of view. This implies that, for people in the poorest segments of the population, nutrition education alone will not be sufficient, and that food aid of good nutritional quality is absolutely needed. This is why specific recommendations are now given to improve the nutritional quality of food aid. **Figure 4.4** shows the structure of food baskets recommended by the French food bank network, based on percentage edible food weights (Rambeloson et al. 2008). By giving priority to meat, fish, vegetables and fruit, they take into account the high cost of these food groups.

Figure 4.4. Recommended composition (in % total weight) of food baskets at French food banks.

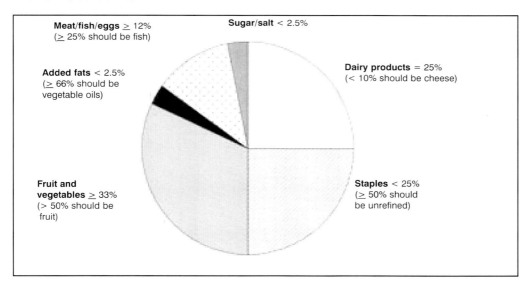

From reference (Rambeloson et al. 2008)

Agriculture Policies

Agriculture policies can be considered the first level of nutrition policy, since they influence farmers' decisions on the kinds and quantities of crops they should grow. Perhaps the most debated agriculture polices in the US are the federal subsidies that are paid to farmers for growing certain crops, which in 2006 amounted to more than 13 billion dollars (Environmental Working Group 2006) and go almost exclusively to four food crops: soy, corn (maize), wheat and rice. Agricultural subsidies that promote grain and oilseed crop production have been said to promote sugars and fats in the food supply, thereby contributing to growing rates of obesity and chronic disease (Wallinga et al. 2009). Economic models indicate that the affordability of most food groups is not due to government subsidies (Miller and Cobie 2007).

A newer area of agriculture policy relates to energy. Growing global demand for energy and dwindling supplies of fossil fuels have caused energy prices to rise and become more volatile. High energy prices can have a direct impact on the cost of food. For instance, high oil prices increase the cost of transporting food long distances to reach the consumer (Edwards and Roberts 2008). Fresh produce prices are particularly vulnerable to rising energy costs as these items are heavy and often require refrigeration during shipping and storage (McLaughlin 2004). Moreover, high prices for fossil fuels have prompted some governments, including the US, to promote alternative energy sources derived from crops. Such policies can have unintended consequences. A period of global inflation in food prices beginning in 2008 was attributed to policies promoting biofuels (Boddiger 2007).

Food Tax and Subsidy Policies

Policies that affect the price of food have the potential to improve the quality of the diet. Food prices can be lowered via subsidies, or raised by the addition of taxes. Food taxes are generally considered a regressive tax policy, since they have a greater impact on the budgets of low-income people than higher-income people. However, there is a growing interest in the use of targeted food taxes to reduce the consumption of less nutritious foods and beverages. Research studies have given inconsistent results. Economic research on the effects of taxes on unhealthy foods suggested that small taxes might have little effect on body weight (Powell and Chaloupka 2009) and might even increase obesity for some people (Yaniv et al. 2009; Schroder et al. 2008). While some studies suggest that taxes might reduce consumption of soft drinks and foods of low nutrient value, and provide revenue to support nutrition of vulnerable groups (Jacobson and Brownell 2000), others have shown that taxes on a single nutrient or a single food tend to have undesired effects on the demand for other nutrients (e.g., fat) or foods (e.g., sweets), due to substitution or income effects (Smed et al. 2007; Mytton et al. 2007).

Alternatively, targeted food subsidies can lower prices for more nutritious foods to make them less costly for consumers. Again, studies have found inconsistent results and even some adverse and unintended consequences. In Egypt, subsidizing bread, wheat flour, sugar, and cooking oil increased the disparity in per calorie costs between energy-dense and energy-dilute foods, which led to increased obesity rates (Asfaw 2006). In a series of community-based intervention studies, researchers found that lowering the price of nutritious foods relative less nutritious food results in an increase in sales of the more nutritious foods (French 2003). Whether such changes in consumption of targeted food items can lead to improvements in the overall diet and in the long term is less clear.

Nutrition Education

Nutrition recommendations for public health, such as those in the *Dietary Guidelines for Americans* (Dietary Guidelines for Americans 2005), the USDA's *MyPyramid* (Center for Nutrition Policy and Promotion), and the cancer prevention food plan from the American Institute for Cancer Research (World Cancer Research Fund 2007) consistently emphasize the need to improve the nutrients-to-energy ratio in the American diet. A large body of research has provided evidence on the health benefits of nutrient dense, low energy density diets (World Cancer Research Fund 2007; Joint

WHO/FAO 2003; Hu and Willett 2002), but there has been less consideration given to the higher monetary cost of such diets.

An important purpose for nutrition education is to highlight the most affordable ways that consumers can achieve dietary recommendations. Since 1975, the United States Department of Agriculture has highlighted affordable nutrition by publishing its Thrifty Food Plan (TFP). The TFP is in essence a prescription for a nutritionally balanced diet at minimal cost. The food plans in the TFP are tailored for age and gender and derived through an optimization process, subject to cost constraints (Becker and Rasmussen 2002). The TFP's optimization achieves relatively low cost in part by including foods that are the least costly sources of important nutrients. The cost of the TFP is revised monthly to reflect retail food prices around the US. The TFP is also periodically revised to reflect changes in dietary guidelines and to take into account changes in the food supply and dietary habits.

The low estimated cost of the TFP is also a result of the assumption that most meals and snacks in the plan are prepared at home from foods bought at supermarkets. In other words, while the TFP might be the lowest-cost way of achieving nutrition recommendations, it might not be convenient. Despite this limitation, the aim of the TFP has been to provide food plans as realistic as possible because those plans are ultimately used for legal and regulatory purposes (Davis and You 2010). Indeed, the Thrifty Food Plan serves as a national standard for a nutritious diet at a minimal cost and is used as the basis for maximum food stamp allotments, and determining poverty thresholds. In essence, the TFP's estimation of a minimum-cost nutritious diet ought to be considered as critical minimum food budget, below which, nutrition education alone would not be helpful in improving diet quality.

More recently, new ways to help consumers identify nutritious and affordable foods have been proposed. Nutrient profiling provides a way to communicate the overall nutritional quality of each food, allowing consumers to relate good nutritional quality to price (Maillot et al. 2007). The concept requires each food to be labelled on the packaging with the nutrient density score, which could help consumers to easily compare foods. For instance, consumers could see that, in many cases, branded products don't have a higher nutritional quality of their low cost equivalents, although their price can be much higher (Darmon et. al 2009; Cooper and Nelson 2003).

Summary and Conclusions

Several lines of evidence indicate that food prices and diet costs present a barrier to a nutritious diet, especially for those of low SES. To understand the relationship between diet quality and diet cost, it is necessary to recognize that there are competing forces acting simultaneously, and depending on their relative strength, various conclusions can be drawn. A low food budget is expected to have an unfavorable impact on diet quality but this impact can be counteracted at least in part by sufficient nutritional knowledge and a motivation to eat healthily. Time and resources too prepare meals are also vital. Thus, it is possible to eat healthily with a low food budget but doing so may involve changing food behaviors and diet patterns dramatically. Indeed, obtaining a low cost nutritious diet may be achieved if particular foods—of high nutrient-to-price ratio—are prioritized. However, such foods might not be typical in the diet, so prioritizing these foods can lead to diets that are nutritious and low cost but less socially acceptable (Maillot et al. 2010). The notion that cost, nutrition and social acceptability are balanced has led some to suggest policy makers, and nutrition professionals should keep in mind the notion that there may be a minimum budget required for a nutritious and socially-acceptable diet.

Footnotes

1) Calculation of milk based on 1,960 grams per half gallon. Calculation of tomatoes takes into account edible portion only.

2) The finding that diets with a high energy cost are both low in energy content and high in nutrients was relatively unexpected. The trend generally seen in nutrition epidemiology is that the more calories people eat the higher are their nutrient intakes. This is just because nutrients do not come alone in foods: they are always associated with dietary energy.

Key Points

1. Foods that are low in energy density and of high nutrient density, such as fruit and vegetables, fish and lean meats are the most expensive sources of dietary energy, whereas foods high in sugar and fats are the least costly ones. The current structure of food prices does not favor the consumption of healthy diets.

2. People living under the poverty level do not have enough money to spend on food, or the dietary changes needed to meet the guidelines at such a cost are not likely to be acceptable, be it on a social or on a behavioral point of view. Economic constraints adversely affect food choices.

3. Obtaining a low cost nutritious diet may be achieved if particular foods—of high nutrient-to-price ratio—are prioritized. Nutrition education might attenuate the negative impact of economic constraints on diet quality.

4. There is a critical minimum food budget, below which, nutrition education alone would not be helpful in improving diet quality. When the budget for food is too low, delivering food aid of good nutritional quality is absolutely needed.

Nutrition Practice Points

When working with clients it is important to consider the client's financial circumstance. With low-income clients, encourage cooking simple meals from scratch as a low cost strategy to stretch the food dollar. Many clients may not have the cooking skills or self-efficacy needed to cook meals from scratch without additional education dedicated to cooking skill development. It is also important to know what food assistance resources are available in your community and how to access those resources; so that you can help your clients utilize those services. You also need to be aware of how your clients feel about food assistance programs and seek to make them more comfortable with using available services. As health professionals we can also play an important role in reducing food insecurity by working with local farm programs, community gardens, and developing social marketing campaigns that seek to change the awareness and perceptions regarding charitable feeding programs. These changes may result in more volunteers and support for charitable feeding programs and greater utilization of the programs by families in need.

Terminology

Disposable income—The money income earned by an individual or household minus taxes on that income (state and/or federal income tax).

Developing countries—Those countries with low level of economic and/or social development, according to objective criteria.

Socioeconomic status—(also Socioeconomic level or socioeconomic position).

Industrialized countries—(also "Developed countries") Those countries with a high level of economic and social development, according to objective criteria.

Food deserts—A term used to describe urban or rural areas that lack food outlets offering nutritious foods.

Food security—The access to enough nutritious food for an active, healthy life. Individuals or households that can not achieve this status are said to be food insecure.

National School Lunch Program—The federally funded National School Lunch Program (NSLP), administered through the USDA's FNS agency, was created in 1946 to provide meal assistance in public, non-profit private schools, and residential child-care institutions.

Nutrient density—A way of expressing the overall nutritional quality of individual foods and total diets. Nutrient density can reflect a number of individual macro- and micro-nutrients contained in foods in relation to their energy content.

Energy density—The amount of energy (in kcal or kJ) per unit weight. Can be used to describe individual foods and total diets.

Food Stamp Program—This federal food assistance program, administered through the U.S. Department of Agriculture's FNS agency, seeks to help families with low incomes eat a healthy diet by providing vouchers for purchasing specific types of foods.

Thrifty Food Plan—Food stamps are provided based on the Thrifty Food Plan (TFP). The TFP is a low-cost diet plan that has been developed by the government and meets the USDA's Dietary Guidelines for Americans. Foods allowed in the plan include breads, cereals, fruits, vegetables, meats, fish, and dairy products. Seeds or plants that produce food are also allowed in the food stamp program. Alcohol, tobacco products, nonfood items, vitamins, medicine, and hot foods are not included for coverage in the food stamp program.

WIC—The Special Supplemental Nutrition Program for Women, Infants and Children is commonly called WIC. This federal program provides supplemental foods, nutrition education, and health care referrals to low-income women who are either pregnant, breastfeeding, or postpartum and to infants and children who are five years old or younger and at nutritional risk.

ACTIVITY

Plan a meal for four people that would meet the Dietary Guideline Recommendations. It should contain a whole grain, fruit, vegetable, lean meat or protein, and a low fat dairy. Go to the store and figure out how much it would cost to make the meal. Also plan a meal for four people that can be whatever you would like. It can be fast and easy. Try to plan for a meal you would really make. Go to the store and figure out how much it would cost to make that meal. Is there a price difference?

Chapter 5

Interpersonal Influences on Food Behavior

Jerica M. Berge and Melissa Nelson Laska

Goal: This chapter examines how interpersonal interactions across the life course influence food behavior.

Objectives: After completing this chapter you should be able to:

1. Identify sources of interpersonal interactions across the life course that may influence food behavior.

2. Describe strategies a parent could adopt to promote their child's healthy eating.

3. Identify potential negative social influences between peers and significant others that may influence food behavior.

4. Understand which interpersonal behaviors may promote healthy eating.

INTRODUCTION

Have you ever considered how your experience of growing up in your particular family influenced the food choices you make? For example, were you a member of the "clean plate club" (being made to finish all of the food on your plate)? Did you have to eat a certain kind of food that you hated? Do you still dislike that food today? When you were sick, was there a certain type of food that your mom cooked to make you feel better? Do you still want that food as an adult when you do not feel good? How many moms fixed a scraped knee or a broken heart over a plate of warm cookies and a cold glass of milk? Why do we have these associations between our image of a "good mom" and homemade chicken noodle soup and warm cookies with milk?

Interpersonal interactions influence our daily and lifetime food behavior. Interactions with people in our lives affect our behavior by influencing social norms, mirrored behaviors, and learned habits. Examining the life course—infancy, childhood, adolescence, young adulthood, adulthood and advanced aging—and the experiences and environments that shape the development of individual's food choices will provide a comprehensive picture of how the interpersonal interactions we are a part of influence our current food behavior (Hetherington 1999).

Infancy

Instantly after a baby is born, one of the first instincts is to eat. Babies are biologically equipped with a rooting reflex (sucking) to help them locate available food and to indicate their need for food to others (Hetherington 1999). The first choice a parent must make regarding the food environment in their child's life is whether to breastfeed or not. Breastfeeding is a practice highly influenced by social norms and social support. In the 1950s breastfeeding was not the social norm and many considered breastfeeding to be "dirty" and less technologically advanced. Through dedicated social marketing and education efforts, the social norms in the United States have been changing. By the 1990s more women were again choosing to breastfeed despite many challenges, such as a dramatic increase in the percent of mothers returning to the work force. However, substantial racial and ethnic disparities in breastfeeding rates still exist, and many women still do not breastfeed, in part because of perceived social norms, workplace settings that are not conducive to breastfeeding and/or lack of social support from friends and family (Bronner, Gross, Caulfield et al. 1999).

When and what solid foods are introduced to children is also greatly influenced by friends and family. Although the nutrition professionals, doctors, and educational literature may recommend the best feeding practices, if a person's friends and family contradict the advised practices and say "this is what we always did" or "this is how it is done," many mothers may make choices based on this social influence instead of medical advice. Strong cultural norms may also impact when and what solid foods are introduced to an infant. For example, previous research suggests that on average low-income African-American mothers may tend to introduce solid foods to their children during very early infancy (earlier than other racial/ethnic and socioeconomic groups), and this is a practice which may very well be supported and encouraged by family and friends (Bronner et al. 1999). Unfortunately, this practice also may be linked with adverse health outcomes for the infant later in life, such as increased risk of developing diabetes (Knip and Akerblom 2005). Significant shifts in cultural and social norms among various racial and ethnic groups are needed in order to promote breastfeeding and other infant feeding practices that are consistent with current health recommendations (American Academy of Pediatrics 2005).

Childhood

Think back to your childhood. Who was it that had an important impact on your eating habits? Most likely it was your parents, family and other people living in your household. Overall, the most influential interpersonal interactions around food behavior in childhood are connected to parent/child dynamics. Children consume roughly three-fourths (75%) of their total calories within the home (Guthrie, Lin and Frazao 2002). Thus, the interpersonal interactions in the home, particularly at meal times, play a major role in the food behavior children adopt. How our parents feed us in early childhood may establish a lifetime of food associations and practices.

Parent Restriction or Control of the Feeding Environment

As children get older, parents utilize varying feeding strategies. Some parents are more controlling or rigid and other parents cater to their children's food desires. As a parent, using pressure or restriction in dealing with a child's eating behavior may be counterproductive to establishing healthy eating patterns. Studies have found that children with mothers who used restriction in feeding during meals were more likely to eat more food and those with mothers who pressured their child to eat during a meal had a greater increase in body mass index (BMI) at age 5-9 (L.L. Birch and Davison 2001).

Parents often use various strategies, such as praise, reasoning, and food as a reward, to encourage their children to increase their food intake. Research has shown that mothers are more likely to use praise to get girls to eat and fathers are more likely to use pressure to get boys to eat more (Neumark-Sztainer 2003; L. L. Birch and Davison 2001; Leann L. Birch 1999; Leann L. Birch and Fisher 1998). Parents who are worried about a child becoming overweight are more likely to restrict consumption of certain foods, rather than pressure the child to eat (May et al. 2007), and be more controlling overall of their child's dietary intake (Berge, Wall, Bauer and Neumark-Sztainer In press; Moens, Braet and Soetens 2007). Over time, however, restrictive parenting with regard to food may paradoxically result in greater levels of eating in the absence of hunger later in life and a greater likely of excess weight gain for the child (Jennifer O. Fisher and Neumark-Sztainer 2003; Neumark-Sztainer 2003). This effect has been demonstrated particularly among girls.

Physiologically, we are made to regulate our own appetite. There are times during growth that children will eat more, and there are times that a child will naturally eat less. It is possible that children who consistently are encouraged to eat more or eat less, without regard to their own appetite, lose the ability to self-regulate intake. Ultimately, it may be important for parents to allow children to regulate their own eating based on satiety cues and hunger levels (L.L. Birch et al. 2001; L.L. Birch and Davison 2001; J.O. Fisher and Birch 1999; L. L. Birch and Fisher 1997; Leann Birch and Fisher 1995;).

Some well-intentioned parents also try to shape the eating patterns of their children by using food as a reward or as a punishment, though generally this is not a recommended practice. Doing so may establish a lifetime of negative emotional eating habits that are related to becoming overweight and/or obese. Many adults may still use food as a reward when they have had a particularly hard day "because they deserve it." This may be a result of childhood experiences involving food reward or punishment strategies used by their family members or teachers. Ideally, parents should offer healthy foods and resist the urge to coerce children to consume more than their bodies tell them to eat. The general guidance, based on the research literature, indicates that the parent should be responsible for providing the healthy food options and the child should be responsible for choosing how much they eat (Rhee, De Lago, Arscott-Mills, Mehta and Davis 2005; L.L. Birch and Davison 2001; L.L. Birch et al. 2001; Leann Birch and Fisher 1995). As a parent, the objective is to simply and consistently offer healthy foods without pressure or creating a power-struggle and allow children to eat when they are hungry. Children will not starve themselves; however, if they have learned that when they reject foods, later they will be offered the foods they are craving, they may continue this pattern.

Parent Modeling of Food Behavior

Parents also promote certain food behavior in children through modeling of food choices. Foods that children see adults eat are more likely to be accepted by children. Parents who have unhealthy eating patterns are more likely to have children with unhealthy eating patterns; and those children are also be more likely to be overweight (K.J. Campbell et al. 2007; L.L. Birch et al. 2001; P.T. Campbell et al. 2001). Research also indicates that mothers who model healthy food choices are more likely to serve more healthy foods, such as fruits and vegetables, to their children and families. Ultimately, the more a child is exposed to a food, and the more they see adults eating that food, the more likely she or he is to like that food. In the long-term, repeated exposure and parental modeling are two positive ways in which parents can promote healthy eating behavior among their children.

Family Meals

Today, it is common to see toddlers drinking sodas and eating a wide array of convenience foods. Children are also more likely to grow up in homes that prepare very few foods from "scratch." Home cooked meals eaten together as a family used to be the norm. However, for many children today, relatively few meals are eaten together as a family and even fewer are prepared at home. Researchers have found that children who eat more meals with their families are more likely to have healthy dietary intake patterns overall, including eating more fruits and vegetables, less fried food and soda, less saturated and trans fat, lower glycemic load, more fiber and micronutrients from food (Fulkerson, Story, Neumark-Sztainer and Rydell 2008; Jacobs and Fiese 2007; L.L. Birch et al. 2001; Davis 1995). Studies have also shown that children who eat meals with their family are less likely to be obese (K.J. Campbell, Crawford and Ball 2006; L.L. Birch et al. 2001; Rosenfield 1988). Overall, family mealtime may yield an important and protective effect for children and adolescents, though the specific mechanism through which family meals impacts health and behavior is poorly understood.

Adolescence

The teenage years represent another unique stage in the lifecourse when interpersonal influences may begin to shift. Although parent influences continue to be important at this age, interpersonal interactions with peers and friends become as important in making food choices as interactions with parents and siblings. As children reach adolescence, they become more autonomous. Parents have less control and peers have a significant influence on food behavior. During this time of emerging autonomy, adolescents are seeking to establish their identity of self. Adolescents often engage in power-struggles and reject parental values or practices. For example, youths may perceive certain foods as foods that their parents would eat; as they reject their parents in the process of developing their identity of self, they may also reject those parent-associated foods. Other foods, often less healthful items such as pizza, soda, and potato chips, may become more socially acceptable among their peer group; as they develop their identity, they may mirror behavior of peers they are consciously or unconsciously trying to become more like. When parents encourage youths to eat more of certain foods, those foods then become less attractive to youths. Conversely, when parents actively seek to restrict certain foods, these foods then become more attractive to adolescents.

Even though adolescents may be seeking more separation from their parents, adolescent's food choices are still influenced by their parents and family during this phase of life. For instance, adolescents consume roughly two-thirds (68%) of their total calories within the home (Guthrie et al. 2002). Home food availability is one of the strongest correlates of eating healthy foods, such as fruits and vegetables, among adolescents (K.J. Campbell et al. 2006; Mary Story and Alton, 1996). Similar to the childhood years, family meal frequency also is associated with greater adolescent intake of fruits, vegetables, grains, and calcium-rich foods, and a lower intake of fried foods, sugar-sweetened beverages, and total fat (Fulkerson et al. 2008; K. J. Campbell et al. 2006; Hanson, Neumark-Sztainer, Eisenberg, Story and Wall, 2005; Neumark-Sztainer, Hannan, Story, Croll and Perry 2003; Neumark-Sztainer, Wall et al. 2003).

Parent Modeling and Encouraging of Food Choices

Modeling and encouraging of both healthy eating and unhealthy eating behavior is of significance when examining adolescents' overall food choice patterns. Research on parental modeling has shown that adolescent's food preferences over time are significantly associated with their mother's food choices, as well as the foods that mothers choose to offer their teenage children (K.J. Campbell et al. 2006; Crawford, Timperio, Tedford and Salmon 2006; Skinner 2002). Other studies have found that parents' encouragement to increase healthy food choices is positively related to healthy dietary intake in adolescent girls and boys (Arcan et al. 2007; K.J Campbell et al. 2006). Furthermore, researchers have also examined the effects of parental encouraging of dieting behavior. These findings have been somewhat counter-intuitive, indicating that adolescents who were encouraged by mothers to diet weigh significantly more than those who were not encouraged to diet. Also, boys who were encouraged to diet were more likely to be worried about gaining weight, currently dieting, and more likely to report unhealthy weight control behavior compared to boys not encouraged to diet (K.J. Campbell et al. 2006). Overall, these results suggest that parents may have a more beneficial impact on their adolescent sons and daughters through modeling healthy food behavior and encouraging healthy food choices, rather than talking about, and focusing on, what they should not eat.

Family Weight Teasing

Unfortunately, social influences can have an extremely detrimental impact on body image and eating patterns, particularly during adolescence, when youth tend to be very aware of their appearance. Research has shown that being teased about weight during adolescence can affect diet-related behavior. Studies have found that family weight-teasing was significantly associated with higher body mass, disordered eating behavior, low body satisfaction, low self-esteem, and high depressive symptoms during adolescence (Eisenberg, Neumark-Sztainer, Haines and Wall 2006; Haines, Neumark-Sztainer, Eisenberg and Hannan 2006; Neumark-Sztainer et al. 2002). Teasing may also have significant long-term effects; another study found that adolescents who were teased by family members about their weight were more likely to be overweight, binge eat, and engage in extreme weight-control behavior five years later (Neumark-Sztainer et al. 2002). Although many families may have the best of intentions, it is estimated that as many as one in every three adolescents has been teased about their weight by their family (Haines et al. 2006; Neumark-Sztainer et al. 2002).

Family Meals

Several studies have found that family meals can have a beneficial impact on youth, not only during childhood but also during adolescence. The frequency of family meals is positively associated with healthy adolescent dietary patterns, including eating more fruits, vegetables, grains, calcium rich foods, protein, calcium, iron, fiber, and drinking fewer soft drinks. Adolescents who eat meals with their family more often are also less likely to engage in unhealthy dieting or extreme weight control behavior (such as vomiting, starvation and taking diet pills) and are less likely to become overweight as older adolescents (Neumark-Sztainer, Eisenberg, Fulkerson, Story and Larson 2008; Jacobs and Fiese 2007; N.I Larson, Neumark-Sztainer, Hannan and Story 2007a; Neumark-Sztainer, Wall, Story and Fulkerson 2004; Neumark-Sztainer, Story, Ackard, Moe and Perry 2000). Researchers have also found that adolescents that have a parent present at the evening meal are more likely to engage in healthy eating patterns (Videon and Manning 2003).

Peer Influences on Food Choices

The relationship between friends and eating patterns has been most thoroughly investigated among adolescent populations. Adolescents who have friends that are dieting or engaging in unhealthy weight control behavior are also more likely to engage in these unhealthy behaviors themselves (Hutchinson, Rapee 2007). Thus, the "type of crowd" youths associate with can have an important influence their own decisions about eating. Youths who associate with the "burnout" crowd have more unhealthy eating patterns and more bulimic behavior. Association with the "brain" crowd is related to healthier eating patterns and increased dieting. Both the "jock" and the "popular" crowd exercise more and the "popular" crowd has an unhealthier eating pattern (Mackey and La Greca 2007). Furthermore, in addition to peer modeling and encouragement to eat certain types of food, peer teasing about one's weight may also have a powerful impact on teens. Similar to family teasing, weight-related teasing among peers has been shown to be associated with disordered eating, low body satisfaction, low self-esteem and depressive symptoms in adolescent populations (Libbey, Story, Neumark-Sztainer and Boutelle 2008; Neumark-Sztainer et al. 2007; Stern et al. 2007; K.J. Campbell et al. 2006).

Young Adulthood

As adolescents become young adults they enter a time of life when for the first time they may be making food choices completely independent of their parents, families and previously established peer networks. The young adult years are marked by important transitions, which may include leaving home, entering college and/or beginning to earn a living. However, despite the fact that this is an age of increased independence in decision-making, many young people at this age may find that other adult responsibilities, such as financial independence and residential and employment stability, are still in flux. Overall, this period of young adulthood is an important, yet understudied, age for establishing health behavior patterns; while these young people are "finding their way in the world" and navigating this confusing time of life, they may also be developing eating patterns that will stick with them for the rest of their lives (Nelson, Story, Larson, Neumark-Sztainer and Lytle 2008).

Research suggests that young adults, on average, have relatively poor dietary intakes (Demory-Luce et al. 2004; Lien, Lytle and Klepp 2001). Findings from national survey data indicate that fast food restaurant use and soft drink consumption is higher among young adults than among any other age group (Nielsen and Popkin 2004; Paeratakul, Ferdinand, Champagne, Ryan and Bray 2003). Furthermore, a majority of young adults consume less than one serving per day of fruit and/or vegetables (Cook and Friday 2005), and report a high frequency of convenience food consumption and "eating on the run"(N.I. Larson, Nelson, Neumark-Sztainer, Story and Hannan 2009). In recent decades, the frequency of family meals and home food preparation among families has declined (Jabs and Devine 2006), leaving many young adults without the skills to prepare foods and plan healthful meals on their own. Overall, the transition from adolescence into the independent living of young adulthood is marked by notable declines in dietary quality that may have important implications for long-term health (N.I. Larson, Neumark-Sztainer, Hannan and Story 2007; Niemeier, Raynor, Lloyd-Richardson, Rogers and Wing 2006; Demory-Luce et al. 2004).

Young adulthood also is a likely time for shifting inter-personal influences and evolving support systems. While the scientific research to support the influence of parents and family on eating-related behavior among children and adolescents is fairly well-established, little research has examined these issues among young adults. Young adults spend more leisure time alone compared to most other age groups (R. Larson 1990) and are often assumed to be somewhat disconnected from their parents and family. However, some research suggests that closer relationships with parents (Aquilino 1997; Thornton, Orbuch and Axxin 1995) and siblings (Scharf, Shulman and Avigad-Spitz 2005) may evolve as youth transition, for example, into college life and through adulthood (Wintre and Yaffe 2000; Berman and Sperling 1991). As youth become more independent, family and social network influences shift; parents may begin to play different roles in the lives of their children, particularly compared to the roles that they served as their children were growing up. Interestingly, the popular press has recently begun to take note of a new segment of parents —dubbed "helicopter parents"—who struggle with the evolution of the parent-child relationship as their children enter young adulthood. These parents hover closely over their children, stay intimately involved in the minute details of their child's life and may even try to inappropriately intervene on their children's behalf in university and/or workplace settings. To date, the prevalence of this "helicopter parenting" is unknown, as is the specific impact of various parenting types of food choices and health behavior during young adulthood. Though it is likely that parents continue to have an important impact on the eating habits of their children throughout young adulthood, additional research is needed to understand the evolving social influences at this age and the extent to which this may influence health behavior patterns.

Overall, young adults face a wide array of barriers to healthy eating. For many young adults, the perception of time scarcity is a dominant feature in their lives, particularly as they try to juggle the demands of school, work, family and/or friends. Previous research also suggests that young adults experience relatively high levels of stress, and many feel as though they do not have adequate stress management skills to cope with the challenges in their life (Nelson, Lust, Story and Ehlinger 2008). This stress may be compounded by numerous other lifestyle factors such as sleep insufficiency, physical inactivity, and/or substance use, all of which increase in prevalence at this age. Research among young adult college students has shown that poor stress management is associated with a wide array of unhealthy lifestyle characteristics, including less physical activity, less fruit and vegetable intake, and less breakfast consumption, as well as increased fast food intake, unhealthy weight control behavior, body dissatisfaction, physical fighting, binge drinking, tobacco use and illicit drug use (Nelson, Lust et al. 2008). Overall, the complex patterning and co-occurrence of risk behavior that occurs particularly during young adulthood may make it challenging for many young people to make healthy choices at this age (Laska, Pasch, Lust, Story and Ehlinger 2009).

Furthermore, emerging adults may feel that they do not have to worry about links between food and long-term disease. Young adulthood is often conceptualized as an age of optimal health and well-being; chronic diseases are often considered something that could happen so far in the future they may not be relevant factors in the current lives of young adults. They may also believe they can make changes in the future to deal with diet and health but that they do not have to worry about it now. Many college students, for example, may be so focused on cramming for the next test, balancing school with work and friends, and seeking romantic partners that behavior associated with long-term disease prevention are not given priority. However, the scientific literature indicates that young adult weight-related behavior (such as eating patterns)—independent of health behavior later in adulthood—may have important implications for both health outcomes during young adulthood, as well as later in life.

Adulthood

As individuals enter adulthood, other major life transitions such as marriage and parenthood become major influences of food choices. Research has indicated that marriage dramatically changes social food interactions. Historically, this was a time when women first began cooking meals independently of their mothers. Many jokes have referenced this as a learning period where many burnt meals are served among newlywed couples. Today, many young couples share cooking responsibilities more equally and many meals are eaten outside of the home.

The influence of peers and social connections are also important in shaping adult eating behavior. Complex social network analysis research has illustrated that a person's chance of becoming obese increases by 57 percent if his or her friend becomes obese. A person's chance of becoming obese only increases by 40 percent when siblings are obese and 37 percent when partners become obese. This relationship is even stronger for friends of the same sex (Christakis and Fowler 2007). Friends who support or sabotage healthy behavior will also influence weight outcomes (Ball and Crawford 2006).

Relationship intimacy may also impact the tone and social context for specific eating occasions. For example, we are more likely to eat more food —particularly less healthful food—when we are with our friends than when we are alone or with strangers (Hetherington, Anderson, Norton and Newson 2006; Clendenen, Herman, Polivy 1994). Perhaps reflecting a long-term consequence of this phenomenon, studies have demonstrated that cohabitation (i.e., sharing a living space with a romantic partner) may be similarly associated with unhealthy behavior changes, perhaps due to changes in the context of eating occasions, as well as the many complexities and life transitions that often accompany cohabitation. Research has shown that young adults who transition from a single or dating relationship to a relationship of cohabitation or marriage are more likely to experience excess weight gain compared to the young adult counterparts who do not experience this life change (Gordon-Larsen 2009).

Another significant time of transition occurs when individuals become parents. There is increased motivation to prepare full, healthy, and balanced meals for their children. As an emerging adult, a person may decide to have ice cream for breakfast and cereal for dinner; however, as parents they may be less likely to let their children have ice cream for breakfast. Although many parents have probably served cereal for dinner on occasion, it is not likely to be an everyday occurrence for most American children. Parents need to consider the impact that their behavior has on the eating patterns of their children; as discussed earlier in this chapter, important parental behavior may include encouragement to eat more or eat less, serving healthy food in the home over repeated exposures, modeling healthy eating behavior, and having family meals frequently.

Advanced Age

As adults age, there are many changes that may affect dietary patterns. Many older adults find their food behavior changes dramatically when they lose their spouse or partner. Many older adults may go through a period of depression after the loss of a spouse that affects food intake. Elderly men, especially, who have had limited experience shopping and preparing their own meals, may have dramatic changes in their food intake patterns when they lose their wife. For anyone who is used to eating meals with someone, the transition to eating alone will affect what and how much is eaten.

Physically, many older adults experience decreased ability to conduct activities of daily living such as shopping, cooking, and cleaning. Taste and smell sensory abilities also deteriorate, affecting the intake patterns of older adults. Deterioration of oral health and/or reductions in digestive functioning that occur with age may also restrict dietary choices. Medications may negatively influence taste, hunger, and satiety. Many older adults have been prescribed restrictive eating patterns to manage chronic diseases. All of these factors may be related to food behavior of older adults.

Summary

From infancy through advanced age our food behavior is influenced by our close relationships and our social interactions. In infancy parents must choose when and how much food they introduce to their children. These decisions can be highly influenced by social norms and family culture/traditions. As children become toddlers and school-aged, parental monitoring of the home food environment has important implications for how children internalize food behavior. Parents who are more controlling or restrictive of the home food environment may create food atmospheres in the home that promote unhealthy eating behavior and weight-related problems in their children. Home environments with frequent family meals, parental modeling of healthy behavior and less weight teasing are more conducive to healthy food behavior such as eating fruits and vegetables and less unhealthy weight control behavior for children and teenagers.

Between the life stages of adolescence and young adulthood food behavior may become more influenced by peers and intimate relationships. Decisions about food behavior are sometimes more influenced by busy schedules and futuristic thinking (e.g., I can change my health behavior later, chronic disease is not an issue for me now). In adulthood, adults become more aware of their own food behavior as many become parents and try to model and provide healthy food choices to their children. Or, when chronic disease becomes more common and they come face-to-face with the consequences of good and bad food behavior. As advanced age becomes a reality, loss of significant others and biological limitations of one's own body influence food behavior. Mental health issues, such as depression and grief/loss, also affect the food choices in later life.

In summary, regardless of what stage of life one is in—infancy, childhood, adolescence, young adulthood, adulthood and advanced aging—food behavior are highly influenced by our interpersonal relationships with others throughout the life course.

Key Points

1. Interpersonal interactions across the life course (infancy, childhood, adolescence, young adulthood, adulthood and advanced aging) have the potential to influence a person's food behavior.

2. Parents need to consistently provide healthy foods, model healthy food behavior, and try to provide as little positive or negative focus on foods as possible.

3. Friends may negatively influence a person's food behavior.

4. Young adulthood is a time of shifting inter-personal influences and evolving support systems, and is an age which individuals may establish life-long behavior patterns.

Nutrition Practice Points

When working with clients, health professionals need to be aware of the complex interpersonal interactions that influence food behavior. Health professionals should take the time to discover the client's social norms and the social norms of the most influential people in the client's life (husband, parents, best friends). When providing information that, if adopted by the client, may present a competing social norm with an influential person in a client's life, health professionals need to be very sensitive and address these potential conflicts. Health professionals can also help clients to identify or find people who could support new positive health behavior.

Terminology

Adolescent—The life stage between childhood and young adulthood, which spans from 13-18 years of age. This time is characterized by multiple changes including, biological, mental, emotional and social.

Adult—The life stage after young adulthood and before advanced age. This stage does not have a particular starting or ending point. One enters adulthood as more responsibilities are taken on in young adulthood and moves into the adult life stage when other transitions such as becoming a parent, getting married, or getting established in a career occur.

Advanced Age—The life stage that occurs when physical decline of the body starts to impede day-to-day activities.

Competing Social Norms—When two different, conflicting social norms exist, and both influence one person, they represent competing social norms.

Childhood—The life stage between infancy and adolescent. Typically between the years of 2-12. During this time the particular stages of childhood are divided further into: (1) toddlers, ages 2-3; (2) preschoolers, ages 4-5; (3) school-aged children, ages 6-10; and (4) 11-12 are pre-adolescents (tweeners).

Feeding Style/Strategies—Behaviors parents use within the home food environment in order to monitor what children eat. For instance, parents may have rules about children eating everything on their plate, they may be restrictive and only allow children to eat certain foods, or they may pressure their child to eat more food.

Young Adulthood—Adulthood does not begin at one single point of time. Instead, a person enters adulthood as he or she begins to take on more responsibilities (life decisions, independent living arrangements, paying bills, etc.) slowly over an extended period of time.

Modeling Behaviors—Dietary behaviors people adopt because they have learned the behavior from another person.

ACTIVITY

- Describe how you interacted with your parents and siblings in relation to food choices as you were growing up.

- Describe friends, and/or significant others who have influenced your food behavior.

- Describe how the interpersonal relationships you are currently in shape the food choices you make now.

- Predict ways in which future major life course changes (e.g. getting married, having children) may affect your food choices.

Chapter 6

Physiology
and Food Behavior

Michael Wheeler and George L. Blackburn

Goal: This chapter introduces you to some physiological factors that influence food behavior.

Objectives: After completing this chapter you should be able to:

1. Identify major areas of hunger and satiety control in the body.
2. Discuss hormones associated with hunger and satiety control.
3. Describe how diet may influence hunger and satiety levels.

Appetite is the desire to consume food based on a number of external cues such as sight, smell, time of day, habits, and social environment. For example, think about one's desire to eat popcorn at the movie theater. Hunger is more narrowly defined as the physiological response indicating a need for food. The hormones that drive hunger are typically released in response to low blood glucose or an empty stomach and trigger our desire to eat. Once we begin to consume food, our sensation of hunger is countered as the feeling of fullness, or satiety, comes. Satiety, like hunger, is controlled by hormones that are released largely from the gastrointestinal tract and brain. It is the balance of these hormones and their corresponding physiological responses that determine when we eat as well as how much we eat. In fact, overeating, referred to as polyphagia or hyperphagia, may be related to a disruption in the regulation of eating behavior-related hormones. The same may be said for a loss of appetite, or anorexia, not to be confused with the mental eating disorder anorexia nervosa.

AREAS OF CONTROL

The gastrointestinal tract, brain, and adipose tissue all function to control energy intake by controlling hunger and satiety. Most of these tissues are capable of producing hormones corresponding to the physiological states of hunger and satiety. The primary region within the brain that responds to and integrates hormone signals is the hypothalamus, which is located just above the brain stem and is about the size of an almond. The hypothalamus, which responds to a wide variety of hormones, can regulate a number of physiological responses such as hunger, thirst, body temperature, anger, immune responses, blood pressure, gastric reflexes, fatigue, and circadian cycles. The hypothalamus connects with the pituitary gland, which links the nervous system to the endocrine system. This hypothalamus-pituitary axis is responsible for many metabolic processes of the autonomic nervous system and hormones that regulate pituitary hormones.

Hormones

The hypothalamus responds to both hunger and satiety hormones that are produced largely by adipose tissue or by the gastrointestinal tract. The predominant afferent hormones, which provide information to the central nervous system, are leptin and ghrelin. Leptin is produced largely by adipose tissue and suppresses hunger. Alternatively, ghrelin is produced mainly by the stomach to stimulate hunger. The hypothalamus as well is capable of producing efferent hormones, signals generated in the brain that carry information to other regions within the brain or away from the brain, which promote hunger or satiety. Several efferent hormones include neuropeptide Y (NPY), agouti-related peptide (AgRP) and melanocyte-stimulating hormone (a-MSH). These and others will be discussed in detail below.

Leptin

Leptin is a hormone that regulates energy intake. It works to decrease appetite and increase metabolism. When leptin was discovered in 1994, many researchers believed it would be the magic bullet to prevent and treat obesity.

Leptin is produced by adipose tissue. The released leptin tells the body that it does not need to eat any more because it has enough energy stored. Leptin signals the body by binding with the appetite center in the brain (the ventromedial nucleus of the hypothalamus) to create a sense of satiety. Generally, as adipose tissue expands due to increased fat storage, it releases more leptin. In fact, most overweight/obese Americans actually have high circulating leptin levels. Leptin then, in theory, should curb eating behavior as people begin to gain weight. However, it was discovered that obese individuals actually suffer from leptin resistance, that is an inability to respond to the leptin signal. This is similar to insulin-resistance in type two diabetes.

The etiology of leptin-resistance is currently unknown. Some researchers suspect that when a person continuously eats beyond the point where the body signals satiety, the receptors that are constantly being bombarded with signals to stop eating may "burn out" and lose the ability to receive the message effectively.

At night, melatonin interacts with insulin to regulate leptin. Inadequate sleep has been associated with increased obesity, possibly in part through the suppression of leptin. Lack of sleep also increases the production of ghrelin.

Ghrelin

Ghrelin is a hormone that stimulates appetite. Ghrelin is produced by the stomach in anticipation of a meal and stimulates increased intake. In some bariatric surgeries, ghrelin is reduced and appetite is reduced. Ghrelin is sensitive to both leptin and insulin. It increases food intake and fat mass through its action on the hypothalamus and activation of neuropeptide Y (NPY). Ghrelin is involved in activation of the mesolimbic cholinergic-dopaminergic reward link. This link serves as a circuit to communicate the reinforcing and hedonic aspects of substances such as foods and addictive drugs (including alcohol). Obese individuals have lower circulating levels of ghrelin. Anorexic individuals have high levels of ghrelin, suggesting that ghrelin seeks to correct imbalances in dietary intake. Prader-Willi Syndrome is a condition associated with increased food intake, BMI, and high levels of ghrelin. Grehlin has also been associated with increased ability to learn and remember things. This suggests that studying on an empty stomach (with subsequent high grehlin levels) may be beneficial to learning.

Gastrin-Releasing Peptide and Cholecystokinin

Both gastrin-releasing peptide (GRP) and cholecystokinin (CCK) are also produced in the gastrointestinal system. Each play a critical role in the digestion of fat and protein. As its name implies, GRP is a hormone that primarily stimultes the release of gastrin, a secondary hormone that stimulates the release of gastric acid secretion. Gastric acid functions to digest food in the stomach. Similarly, CCK is a hormone that aids in the digestion and absorption of fat and protein. CCK is also related to feelings of satiety. It is proposed that CCK opposes the effects of ghrelin. Whether or not CCK has a neurological effect is still an area of research. One hypothesis is that the CCK reduces hunger by delaying gastric emptying. It is also of interest, that CCK has a larger satiety effect in males than females.

Obestatin

Other hormones related to hunger and satiety have recently been discovered. Obestatin is a hormone discovered in 2005 that is encoded by the pre-proghrelin gene that also encodes for ghrelin. Surprisingly, however, obestatin appears to have the opposite effect of ghrelin as it functions to decrease appetite. Obestatin is of interest since it also reduces fluid intake through its actions on the brain's thirst center.

Orexins

Orexins (or hypocretins) are hormones predominantly produced by hypothalamic neurons that project throughout the central nervous system to cells involved in feeding control, sleep/wake behavior, and addictive behavior. In regards to their relation to food intake, orexins stimulate hunger (increase craving for food) and energy expenditure. Interestingly, orexin-positive neurons have been discovered to project into the gastric fundus and are thought to control gastrointestinal motility. Initial research on orexins—Orexin-A and Orexin-B—was heavily focused on their role in appetite regulation. However, these peptides have also been shown to influence a wide variety of other physiological and behavioral processes, including wakefulness, locomotor activity and pain thresholds.

Neuropeptide Y and Melanocyte-Stimulating Hormone

Leptin also functions in hunger regulation by inhibiting neuropeptide Y (NPY) and agouti-related peptide (AgRP) and increasing expression of melanocyte-stimulating hormone (α-MSH). NPY stimulates hunger and α-MSH increases satiety. NPY is a neurotransmitter found in the brain. In addition to stimulating hunger, NPY is also associated with memory, learning, increasing fat stores, and decreased physical activity. Stress, high fat intake, and high sugar intake are associated with increased levels of NYP and increased fat accumulation in the abdomen.

Corticotropin-Releasing Hormone

Corticotropin-releasing hormone (CRH) is associated with NPY and leptin. CRH is associated with decreasing hunger and increasing physical activity. CRH is a hormone produced in the paraventricular nucleus (PVN) (a part of the hypothalamus) in response to stress.

DIET AND SATIETY

The food we eat also influences our hunger and satiety. Fiber intake, which increases CCK and provides bulk, is associated with increased satiety. Fat also increases satiety and delays stomach emptying, thereby increasing time between feelings of hunger. Fat also results in a blunted glucose spike in reaction to carbohydrate intake. If glucose levels in the blood rapidly increase and drop, this may result in increased hunger and food craving. Mixed meals (carbohydrate, fat, and protein) result in a blunted blood glucose response. The increase in blood glucose levels from ingestion of carbohydrate-containing food is measured by the glycemic index. Dehydration may also send signals that can be misinterpreted as hunger cues. Water in the stomach consumed prior to a meal may decrease the food intake at the subsequent meal.

The evidence that dietary protein influences the satiety/hunger balance is extensive. Dietary protein increases CCK secretion, which delays gastric emptying and suppresses the effects of ghrelin. Dietary protein may directly or indirectly alter the balance of NPY and POMC in the hypothalamus. Some evidence suggests that leucine, an amino acid derived from a high protein diet, may function to suppress NPY neurons. Clearly, the evidence that laboratory animals fed high protein diets eat less is convincing.

The Senses

Our senses also play a role in hunger. Smell in particular is intrinsically associated with taste. Smell and taste both affect food consumption. There are five different tastes: sweet, sour, salty, bitter, and savory. If people have reached satiety with foods that have a specific taste profile, they may still experience hunger and craving for different tastes. This is why so many people, even when they are stuffed after a meal, can still find room for dessert. The preference for sweet is also a biological drive. Even infants are born with a preference for sweet things. Infants will make positive faces and seek out sweet tasting liquid and make negative reactions to bitter liquids and reject second tastes. Taste may also be genetically influenced. The same individuals who are more likely to be sedentary may also be more likely to physiologically crave sweets and fats. Some individuals have very highly developed palettes (supertasters) and require less food to reach sensory satisfaction. Some individuals may have less sensitive taste receptors (non-tasters) and require more food (highly salted or sweet) to reach a similar level of satisfaction. As individuals age, they may experience decreased ability to smell and taste that can result in decreased intake of food.

Key Points

1. Hunger and satiety are controlled in the body by the brain, gastrointestinal tract, and adipose tissue.
2. Hormones associated with hunger and satiety control include leptin, ghrelin, NPY, obestatin, nesfatin-1, melanocyte stimulating hormone, agouti-related peptide, corticotrophin-releasing hormone, orexin, gastrin-releasing peptide, and cholecystokinin.
3. Fiber, fat, and protein will extend the sensation of fullness.

Nutrition Practice Points

When working with clients, health professionals need to be aware that physiology may be playing a significant role in clients' hunger and satiety levels, their success in dieting, and what foods they crave. Although current science does not provide effective therapies to address many of these hormonal influences on food behavior, it is important for health professionals to stay current on research and be prepared to help clients understand future therapies that may become available. It is also helpful for health professionals to recognize and discuss these biological drives and impairments with clients and the fact that without current therapies available all we can do is modify behavior. Acknowledging the physiological struggles that clients may be facing may help them accept the realities of needed behavior changes.

Terminology

Anorexia—Lack of appetite.

Anorexia Nervosa—An eating disorder where individuals have a severely disordered view of their body weight and seriously restrict calorie intake producing very low body weight.

Agouti-related Peptide—A neuropeptide produced in the hypothalamus that increases appetite and decreases physical activity.

Autonomic Nervous System—Part of the peripheral nervous system; it functions to keep the body in automatic homeostasis. It acts as the control system for the body regulating multiple processes essential for life including breathing, heart rate, perspiration, and many other functions.

Corticotropin-releasing hormone—A neurotransmitter released by the hypothalamus in response to stress that decreases hunger and increases physical activity.

Cholecystokinin—A peptide hormone released by the gastrointestinal tract that increases satiety.

Endocrine System—A collection of small organs that function to release and control hormones in the body.

Gastrin-releasing Peptide—A hormone produced in the stomach that functions in the digestion of food.

Gastrointestinal tract—A system of organs including (mouth, pharynx, esophagus, stomach, small intestines, large intestines, and anus) that functions to take in, digest, and absorb food and expel food waste products.

Ghrelin—A hormone produced by the stomach and the pancreas that stimulates appetite.

Hormone— Chemicals released by cells that affect other cells. They are the body's messengers.

Hypothalamus—Almond shaped and located just above the brain stem, the hypothalamus is the link between the nervous system and the endocrine system through the pituitary gland. The hypothalamus controls many functions of the autonomic nervous system and metabolic processes. It controls body temperature, anger, thirst, fatigue, hunger, and circadian cycles.

Leptin—A hormone produced by adipocytes that tells the brain to stop eating. However, many obese individuals have high levels of leptin without reduced hunger because of leptin-insensitivity.

Melanocyte Stimulating Hormones—Produced in the hypothalamus, these hormones control the melonocytes of the hair and skin (pigmentation/color). In the brain it also stimulates satiety.

Melatonin—A hormone that helps to set the body's natural clock (circadian rhythm).

Non-tasters—People who have a decreased ability to taste. Non-tasters may seek more food, sweeter food, or saltier food to compensate for the lack of taste they experience.

Neurpeptide Y—A neurotransmitter in the autonomic nervous system and brain that increases food intake and decreases physical activity.

Nesfatin-1—A protein in the brain that decreases hunger, food intake, and body fat.

Obestatin—A peptide hormone produced by the cells that line the gastrointestinal tract (specifically the stomach and small intestines) and functions to decrease appetite.

Orexin—A pair of neuropeptide hormones, called orexins or hypocretins, that stimulate food intake, wakefulness, and energy expenditure.

Paraventricular Nucleus—A grouping of neurons in the hypothalamus that produce hormones.

Peptide—Chains of amino acids are called peptides because the link between the amino acids is a peptide bond.

Pituitary Gland—A pea-sized endocrine gland that produces many hormones and is located in the brain at the bottom of the hypothalamus.

Polyphagia (or hyperphagia)—Eating too much or increased eating.

Satiety—Feeling full and lacking hunger.

Super-tasters—People who can taste very acutely and are more sensitive to some specific types of tastes.

Ventromedial Nucleus—The nucleus (or center) of the hypothalamus; it has a role in satiety.

ACTIVITY

Keep a food diary for one day. Write down what foods and what time you eat. Also write down how hungry you feel throughout the day. Do you see any relationship between the times and types of foods you ate and the times that you were hungry?

Chapter 7

Cultural Influences on Food Intake Behavior

Nurgul Fitzgerald, Susan Gabriel,
and David Himmelgreen

Goal: This chapter introduces you to acculturation and its influence on food intake-related behaviors.

Objectives: After completing this chapter you should be able to:

1. Define acculturation.
2. Identify the linkages between acculturation and food- and lifestyle-related behaviors.
3. Discuss nutrition education strategies that can be used when working with immigrants.

There are more than 150 definitions of culture (Kroeber and Kluckholn 1952). Yet, one definition that has stood the test of time is provided by the 19th Century anthropologist Edward Tylor who wrote that culture is the "complex whole that includes knowledge, belief, art, morals, law, custom, and any other capabilities and habits acquired by man as a member of society" (Tylor 1924). In other words, culture is a set of attitudes, beliefs, and values that are shared and accepted among members of a group or community. We often identify cultural background by ethnicity, country of origin, religious affiliation, commonly shared ideals, or by a community with commonly shared characteristics or behaviors. These cultural characteristics are also reflected in food-related behaviors and can ultimately influence the overall health status. This chapter will present an overview of the associations between acculturation and food intake-related behaviors and provide suggestions for appropriate nutrition education approaches. Because Hispanics are the largest immigrant or minority population in the United States (US), examples of these associations among Hispanics will be highlighted.

ACCULTURATION

Acculturation can be defined as "the process by which immigrants adopt the attitudes, values, customs, beliefs, and behaviors of a new culture" (Abraido-Lanza 2004). Although communities and societies also change by the influence of individuals, the majority of the studies about acculturation in the literature usually refers to the changes that individuals or immigrants go through while they become accustomed to the characteristics of the newer culture. Acculturation is a multidimensional process, and individuals can be classified into several categories within this process. Some examples of these categories include: assimilated (completely adapted to the newer culture and lost the traits of the culture of origin), marginalized (exclusion by both cultures), separated or segregated (retained the traits of the culture of origin without integrating into the newer culture), and integrated or bicultural (accepted both cultures) (Perez-Escamilla and Putnik 2007; Lara, Gamboa et al. 2005). It should be noted that care must be taken when attempting to categorize an individual based on his/her level of acculturation because of the potential for ethnic stereotyping (Hunt, Schneider et al. 2004) and a blaming the victim mentality where the person is faulted.

Although many categories within the acculturation continuum exists, sometimes it can be difficult to determine these stages because of the need to use comprehensive scales to appropriately measure several dimensions of acculturation. Limitations in time and other resources often force researchers to use shorter measures of acculturation. Commonly used acculturation measures almost always include questions about the language use (e.g., language used to think, at home, or with friends). Additionally, researchers sometimes use individual questions such as language spoken at home, length of residence in the country or generational status (e.g., country of birth, first versus second generation in the country) as a proxy of acculturation status (Lara, Gamboa et al. 2005).

As a result of these various measures of acculturation, reports of the potential impact of acculturation on food intake and health can be mixed. One must also keep in mind that acculturation can bring about both positive and negative influences on food- and health-related behaviors, and these influences might vary based on the characteristics of the newer culture and the culture of origin.

Dietary Acculturation

Similar to general acculturation, dietary acculturation can be defined as the process by which immigrants adopt the food-related beliefs, values, attitudes, and dietary intake behaviors of the host culture. This process is "multidimensional, dynamic, and complex; [and] varies considerably, depending on a variety of personal, cultural, and environmental attributes" (Satia-Abouta, Patterson et al. 2002). The influence of acculturation on dietary intake is not the same for all ethnic groups. However, less acculturated individuals usually tend to show healthier dietary intake patterns in comparison to their more acculturated counterparts in the US (Ayala, Baquero et al. 2008; Lara, Gamboa et al. 2005). For example, an analysis of the national data from the National Health and Nutrition Examination Survey (NHANES 1999-2004) revealed that foreign-born Hispanic adults reported consuming more fruits, vegetables, fruit and vegetable juices, and high-fiber/low-fat breads, and less snacks, desserts, soda, fruit drinks, and fast foods than their US-born counterparts (Duffy, Gordon-Larsen et al. 2008).

Other studies suggest that less (versus more) acculturated Mexican Americans have a higher diet quality that adheres more closely to the dietary recommendations in the United States. For example, it has been reported that Mexico-born or first generation Mexican Americans consume less fat, and more fiber, protein, vitamins A, C, E and B6, folate, calcium, potassium, and magnesium than their US-born or second generation counterparts (Dixon, Sundquist et al. 2000; Guendelman, Abrams et al. 1995). These differences in nutrient intake might be because of less acculturated Hispanics' greater consumption of fruits, vegetables, whole grains, legumes, traditional Mexican foods (e.g., corn tortillas, beans, rice), and unsaturated fats, and less consumption of desserts, sugar, sugar-sweetened beverages, and added fats (e.g., salad dressing, butter/margarine, mayonnaise) (Ayala, Baquero et al. 2008; Neuhouser, Thompson et al. 2004; Dixon, Sundquist et al. 2000; Bermudez, Falcon et al. 2000; Romero-Gwynn et al. 1993).

With regard to acculturation, parental feeding practices are also worth consideration. Worrying about children being underweight and using food to calm children have been reported to be more common among Spanish-speaking Hispanics than English-speaking Hispanics in the US (Evans, Greenberg et al. 2009). Because children's food preferences are established early and greatly affected by what is made available to them by their parents, the influence of acculturation on parental feeding practices can set the stage for the eating patterns of children in the future.

Causes of Dietary Change

Availability and cost of foods have been reported among the reasons for changes in immigrants' dietary patterns (Satia, Patterson et al. 2000). It must be noted that insufficient availability of traditional foods in the US may be undergoing a change as the number of immigrants and public interest in various ethnic cuisines continue to increase. Parallel to the growth in the various ethnic groups (e.g., Latinos), more and more supermarkets are making available an increasing number of ethnic foods, and many small stores targeting specific segments of population are able to provide such traditional food products. Thus, availability may not be the same barrier to continuing a traditional ethnic diet pattern it once was.

Availability and cost can be barriers for healthful food habits in other ways. Decreased availability of a variety of fresh and low-cost fruits and vegetables, and increased availability of low-cost processed high-fat and/or high-calorie foods (e.g., fast foods) can change individuals' food choices. These characteristics are commonly seen especially in socioeconomically disadvantaged urban areas, and acculturation towards this lifestyle in such environments can negatively influence immigrants' food intake patterns as these new foods replace potentially healthier traditional foods.

Changes in food intake through the acculturation process can vary based on the cost and availability of foods in the US as well as the country of origin. For example, higher cost and less availability of certain foods, such as fresh fruits or traditional Mexican foods, and lower cost and increased availability of snacks, sweets, and fast foods in the US have been reported as reasons for changes in eating behaviors among Hispanics (Colby 2009; Himmelgreen 2007; Gray 2005). Additionally, it has been reported that some foods, such as mayonnaise, margarine, and salad dressing, were considered high-status items by many low-income families in Latin America possibly because of cost and availability issues (Romero-Gwynn et al. 1993). Similarly, in a qualitative study of pre- and post-migration dietary changes, Colombian adults living in Florida reported that in addition to fast food not being as readily available in their native country, it was more expensive than in the US. Therefore, people tended to eat fast food only for special occasions, such as birthdays, in their native country (Himmelgreen, Romero Daza et al. 2007). Lower costs and wide availability of these foods in the US are likely to result in increased consumption.

Despite these differences, one must also take into account that food environment continues to change in Mexico or other countries as well as in the US. Availability of highly processed foods, sugary drinks, and fast food is on the rise in many countries outside the United States, and depending on what was available in the location of origin, immigrants might be increasingly facing similar food choices in their home countries and in the US. Therefore, although immigrants are generally more likely to have healthier food intake patterns in their home countries, it may also be wrong to make such an assumption without asking them about their past and current intake patterns.

In addition to the cost of foods, overall economic abilities of individuals also affect their food choices. Immigrants and minorities usually are more likely to have a lower socioeconomic status and to suffer from food insecurity (Nord, Andrews et al. 2009). Such economic limitations are likely to force individuals to purchase relatively cheaper and filling but often nutrient-poor, energy-dense foods, which can lead to obesity (Townsend 2009; Rosas 2009; Drewnowski 2005).

Work schedules or busier lifestyles are other factors influencing food choices of families in the US. Mexican immigrants report that in comparison to the more relaxed lifestyle in Mexico, there is a more scheduled lifestyle, including after-school obligations and planned events, and less time to cook in the US, and this type of lifestyle results in an increase in their fast food consumption (Colby, Morrison et al. 2009; Gray, Crossman et al. 2005).

It is also very important, especially when working with first generation immigrant families, to recognize the role of children as the primary drivers of the family's acculturation process because parents report that their children influence the food purchasing decisions in the household (Gray, Crossman et al. 2005). Dietary acculturation can be a detrimental process for immigrant youth who are developing self and ethnic identity, and seeking separation from their parents and acceptance from their peers (e.g., to be more like other kids at school). For example, in their efforts to become a part of the new culture, children may identify fast foods and other less healthful food options with the culture of the United States, may change their eating patterns (Gray, Crossman et al. 2005), and subsequently influence their families' food intake decisions. Reports suggest that one of the biggest changes in children's diets after moving to the US occurs with the foods they eat at school; children still like the traditional Mexican foods they receive at home, but they prefer the American foods they are served at school (e.g., pizza, hamburgers) (Colby, Morrison et al. 2009; Gray, Crossman et al. 2005). Furthermore, Mexican-American youth have reported not believing there to be any differences in the healthfulness of traditional Mexican diets (they defined it as fruits, vegetables, and beans) versus the American diet, which they defined as hotdogs, hamburgers, French fries, and pizza (Colby, Morrison et al. 2009).

Exposure to food and beverage advertisements through a variety of media outlets in the US can also stimulate changes in dietary intake patterns of children and their families. Research has shown that children choose the advertised foods at significantly higher rates and attempt to influence the food purchasing decisions of their parents (Chamberlain 2006; Halford 2004; Story 2004). Because types of foods most often advertised on television are nutritionally poor and energy-dense (e.g., high sugar cereals, candy, soft drinks, chips) (Kunkel, McKinley et al. 2009), children and their families are most likely to be negatively influenced from ongoing exposure to such influence. Advertisements of these nutritionally inferior food choices are widespread through a variety of channels such as schools (vending machines, corporate sponsorship of school events and materials, etc.), and online applications (e.g., interactive games, sweepstakes, computer screensavers, etc.). Therefore, educating immigrant parents and children about these potential media influences, risks of certain American dietary intake patterns (higher fat, added sugar, and calories) and benefits of the traditional healthy dietary habits from their culture of origin become important issues to address in relationship to dietary acculturation.

Acculturation, Lifestyle, and Disease Risk

Previous sections highlighted the potential changes in dietary intake patterns as individuals acculturate. Dietary intake is related to many health conditions and chronic diseases such as obesity, type 2 diabetes, and cancer. In addition to food intake, other lifestyle factors (e.g., physical activity, media use) are also likely to be influenced by the acculturation process and may lead to further variations in disease risks immigrants might face. Moreover, socioeconomic status of immigrants is often more compromised in comparison to non-immigrants, and this can also influence food intake, lifestyle and other health-related behaviors, and susceptibility to chronic diseases.

Obesity is linked to increased risk for several chronic diseases including some cancers and type 2 diabetes (World Cancer Research Fund 2007; Field 2001), and studies suggest that more acculturated individuals have higher rates of obesity compared to less acculturated individuals in the US. Popkin and Udry reported that second or third generation Hispanic youths were more likely to be overweight than those who were the first generation in the US (Popkin and Udry 1998). For adults, Goel (Goel, McCarthy et al. 2004), Fitzgerald (Fitzgerald, Himmelgreen et al. 2006), and Himmelgreen (Himmelgreen, Perez-Escamilla et al. 2004) also reported that highly acculturated Latinos—as determined by length of residence or language use—were more likely to have higher BMIs than their less acculturated counterparts (Abraido-Lanza, Chao et al. 2005; Crespo, Smit et al. 2001). These reports point out the importance of nutrition and lifestyle interventions to prevent obesity among minorities such as Latinos.

In addition to the rates of obesity, physical activity levels also differ by acculturation status. Because immigrants and minorities are more likely to have a low socioeconomic status, they may have more physically demanding jobs or be more physically active for the necessities of everyday living (e.g., walking to/from bus stop or grocery stores because of not owning a car). However, studies suggest that highly acculturated Hispanics in the US are more likely to be physically active during leisure-time than their less acculturated counterparts. This might be a reflection of better socioeconomic conditions that highly acculturated individuals may achieve. As a result of better education and greater exposure to health-related information and services, highly acculturated individuals may value and be able to successfully change their behaviors towards healthier options. With better economic resources, they would be more likely to overcome barriers such as lack of transportation or costs associated with after-school organized sports, fitness centers or clubs, and concerns about neighborhood safety.

Aforementioned findings point out that acculturation is linked to food intake and related health conditions and lifestyle behaviors, such as obesity, socioeconomic conditions, and physical activity. It is important to remember that all of these factors are also linked to chronic diseases like cancer or type 2 diabetes and present as important aspects in promoting health among minorities in the United States.

NUTRITION PRACTICE POINTS

As explained in the previous sections, acculturation is an important aspect of individuals' food intake and lifestyle behaviors. When providing services, nutrition professionals need to adapt the assessment, education, and counseling strategies to meet the individual's unique stage of acculturation and be effective in promoting healthier lifestyles.

During an initial assessment of an immigrant's diet, it is important to ask some questions to better understand the individual's cultural perspectives, which may influence his or her behavior. Being respectful, open to and accepting of other individuals' cultural or ethnic differences and then developing a sense of trust and rapport are the first and most essential steps a health professional must take when working with immigrants. Prior knowledge of various ethnic and cultural characteristics for communication, foods, and food-related behaviors are necessary to be able to build this rapport and trust. Once rapport is established, some of the following questions may be helpful to have an idea about the acculturation status of the individual (in this case, assumed to be a Mexican American):

1. Where were you born? If born in the United States: where were your parents born? If born in Mexico: how many years have you been in the United States?
2. What language do you mostly speak at home (mostly/only Spanish, mostly/only English, or Spanish and English equally)?
3. Do you watch mostly or only Spanish TV, mostly or only English TV or both equally?
4. What language do you usually speak with your friends (mostly/only Spanish, mostly/only English, or Spanish and English equally)?

5. What types of foods do you usually eat (mostly/only Mexican foods, mostly/only American foods, or Mexican and American foods equally)?

   Although the questions like the ones listed above are helpful to determine a general reference point regarding individuals' acculturation levels, it is also important to remember that each individual might be very unique. A person who has been in the United States for 40 years may be acculturated very little towards the mainstream American culture. That is why it is important to use these questions as general guidelines rather than absolute measures of various acculturation levels.

   Individuals will respond best to nutrition education that is tailored to meet their acculturation status. Some examples of different nutrition education or counseling approaches depending on various acculturation stages are given below:

   - **Individuals who identify mostly or only with their culture of origin** (e.g., Mexican American, moved to the US as an adult, speak mostly or only Spanish, and prefer mostly or only Mexican foods): They are likely to benefit from encouragement to continue following healthy traditional food intake patterns from their primary culture and may need to be made aware of the risks associated with some of the American dietary intake patterns.

   - **Individuals who self-identify with both cultures equally** (e.g., Mexican American, moved to the US as an adult, speaks both languages equally, eats both Mexican and American foods equally): Emphasizing the benefits of healthful traditional Mexican food intake patterns will be useful to help them maintain these patterns since it is easier to retain the existing food habits than adjusting to new habits. Additionally, the healthier food options from the American cuisine must be emphasized to prevent the adoption of unhealthful food intake habits.

   - **Individuals who identify mostly with American culture** (Mexican American, moved to the US as a child or was born in the US, speaks both languages but mostly English, and prefers American foods most of the time): It would probably be easier for these individuals to make adjustments to their existing (American) dietary patterns to select the healthier food options rather than suggesting them to go back to their ethnic traditional food intake patterns. However, it may still be useful to raise awareness about the healthfulness of some of their traditional (Mexican) food patterns if they, at times, still prefer such foods. Considering that more people everyday take pride in their ethnic backgrounds, and they try to incorporate their ethnic past into their current lifestyles, emphasizing these healthier traditional foods would be an excellent opportunity for successful behavior change in this case.

As mentioned earlier, hardly anyone will completely fall into one particular stage of acculturation by just using the number of years they resided in the US or the language they speak. The important point is to take each individual's cultural behavior patterns into account and find a reasonable solution *working together* with that individual. The overall goal is to find the comfort level of each person in terms of specific food-related behaviors and help him or her make gradual adjustments toward eating more healthfully while staying within the limits of what is familiar and acceptable to that person.

Nutrition messages that promote healthful traditional eating patterns can be empowering in that they celebrate and recognize the strengths of an immigrant's cultural background. If health promotion programs promote non-ethnic American food choices to newly arrived immigrants, then they ask the immigrants not only change to a new cultural eating pattern, but they also ask to make the healthier choices within that new pattern that are usually not supported by the existing food environment in the US. Therefore, success would be an unlikely outcome with this approach. By encouraging the retention of healthful and culturally appropriate foods that are already familiar, there may be an opportunity to make a significant impact on the health of a growing proportion of our nation's population.

Key Points

1. Acculturation is associated with changes in dietary intake patterns and other lifestyle behaviors (e.g., physical activity). These changes are likely to influence the risk for obesity and chronic diseases including cancer and type 2 diabetes.

2. Care must be taken when attempting to categorize an individual based on his/her level of acculturation because of the potential for ethnic stereotyping. Although there are some questions that help determine the acculturation status, nutrition education and counseling should be tailored to the specific food behavior characteristics of each individual and should include their active participation.

3. It is beneficial for immigrants to maintain their healthful traditional dietary practices from their culture of origin.

4. It is important to raise awareness among immigrants about the less healthful food options and to have them develop the skills in adopting the healthier food intake patterns in the United States.

Terminology

Acculturation—The process by which immigrants adopt the attitudes, values, customs, beliefs, and behaviors of a new culture.

Dietary acculturation—The process whereby an individual from one culture comes into a new culture and subsequently adopts the new culture's food-related beliefs, values, attitudes, and dietary intake behaviors.

ACTIVITY

Pick a location culturally different from your own and learn as much as you can about that place. Seek opportunities to talk to people from that area and try foods traditional to that culture.

Determine what aspects of these foods would be healthful choices or how they can be modified toward being more healthful while remaining culturally acceptable.

Chapter 8

Changing Food Intake Patterns: Health Behavior Theories

Carol Byrd-Bredbenner and Virginia Quick

An important goal of health and nutrition professionals is to help consumers gain the knowledge, skill, desire, and motivation needed to adopt healthier behaviors. Much of this help is provided via communication. These communications may be written, oral, or a combination of the two (Table 1). When developing nutrition communications for consumers, it is important to think about "why" consumers select the foods they do as well as "how" behavior change occurs. Keeping the how and why in mind maximizes the chances that communications will equip and motivate individuals to improve their health by modifying their behaviors.

Table 1. Communication Methods

Form	Examples
Written	newspapers, magazines, newsletters, books, pamphlets, brochures, factsheets, texting, websites, blogs
Oral	radio, podcasts, CDs, phone calls
Written and Oral Combined	television, movies, DVDs, webinars

Why Do Consumers Eat the Foods They Do?

The most important factors affecting food choices are food appeal, health considerations, and economics (Table 2). Food appeal includes taste, food appearance, and preferences. Nearly all research identifies taste as the most important factor affecting food choices [1-8].

Health considerations include food safety, nutrition (nutrients in food), and weight control (calories in food). When it comes to selecting foods, most consumers, especially females, rate the importance of health considerations very close to taste [7, 8]. Although adults of all ages report that nutrition is an important factor when making food choices [7, 9-11], its importance is rated higher by older adults [1] and lower by teens [2]. Concern about body weight, physical appearance, and attractiveness guides food selection for many people and may be a more important motivator than overall health [11, 12]. One national study reported that weight control concerns were most important to older people [1] and another reported that among college students, weight concern is the most common reason given for actively avoiding certain foods [13].

Economic considerations include the monetary cost of food as well as the time and effort needed to obtain, prepare, and eat food. Food price is important to most adults, but its level of importance generally trails far behind taste, food safety, and nutrition [7]. Younger people, women, and low income individuals rate food cost and the need for convenient, easy preparation as more important than other groups [1, 7, 9, 10, 14]. Adults of all ages, especially young adults living alone, report that lack of time greatly influences their food choices. Today, more than 40% of dinners prepared at home are ready to eat in less than 30 minutes (Figure 1) [15]. Lack

Figure 1: Sandwiches are the most popular dinnertime main dish [19]

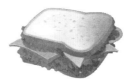

of food preparation skills and disinterest in food preparation activities are other factors affecting food choices [16-18], such as frequent use of convenience foods, take-out foods from restaurants and supermarkets, and no cook meals [15, 19].

Table 2. Key Factors Affecting Food Choices

Factor	Examples
Food Appeal	Taste, Food Appearance, Food Preferences
Health	Food Safety, Nutrition, Weight Control
Economics	Food Cost, Time and Effort to Obtain, Prepare, and Eat Food
Other	Nutrition Knowledge and Skills, Food Marketing, Familiarity, Novelty, Cultural and Ethical Considerations, Environmental Issues, Food Ingredient Concerns, Religious Doctrine, Situation or Occasion, Associative Meanings

Some other factors that affect food choice include knowledge and marketing. Knowledge about food and nutrition may influence food choices [20-22]. For example, in one study, participants with the most nutrition knowledge were nearly 25 times more likely to meet fruit, vegetable, and fat intake recommendations than those with the least knowledge [22]. Food marketing, including advertising, can affect food choices particularly those made by children [23]. Several studies report that marketing affects nutrition knowledge and beliefs [24-26], increases the number of and type of food children request and choose [27-30], and increases snacking frequency as well as calorie and nutrient intake [31-33].

Other factors that may shape food choices are familiarity (preference for foods they have eaten before), novelty (desire to be adventurous and try new foods), ethical considerations (concern about global warming, animal rights), environmental issues (desire to avoid certain contaminants, pesticides), food ingredients (desire to avoid certain ingredients, like food additives or allergens or eat certain ingredients, such as soy), religious doctrine (desire to comply), situation or occasion (mood, people individuals are eating with, traditional foods eaten on certain occasions), and associative meanings (comfort, memories) [3, 6, 15, 34-38]. However, these other factors are not yet well studied.

Many people do not realize a nutritious diet can be composed of foods that are appealing, healthy, economical, and fulfill other important personal preferences and goals, such as those related to ethics, environment, or religion. The challenge for nutrition professionals is to help consumers realize how they can "have it all." That is, show them how they can change (improve) their diets (and health!) using foods with the qualities that are important to them.

HOW DOES BEHAVIOR CHANGE OCCUR?

In the last 60 years, researchers have developed theories to help us understand why people behave the way they do and how health professionals can help them change their behavior. A **theory** is a set of related constructs that explain why an event (behavior) has occurred or predict how an event (such as behavior change) will occur. (Note that the terms "theory" and "model" often are used interchangeably.) **Constructs**, also called concepts, are the major ideas or building blocks of a theory [39]. As you will see below, a theory's constructs could include a person's knowledge, attitudes, confidence that he or she can perform a behavior, or other factors. A drawing often is developed to show how constructs in a theory are organized and related to each other, such as you will see later in Figure 5. The most useful theories tell a logical, clear "story" that accurately reflects the factors affecting health behaviors.

Strong research evidence indicates that health and nutrition behavior change proceeds through a series of stages. Several stage-based theories have been developed to describe the steps that people follow as they try to change a health behavior. Although these theories differ in the number and description of stages, all have three main steps starting with "preintention" (i.e., not planning to perform a particular behavior) then moving on to intention (i.e., deciding to perform a particular behavior, but not performing it yet) and finally action (i.e., actually performing a behavior) [40, 41]. See Figures 2 and 3. The goal of nutrition communicators is to help consumers move through these stages and ultimately, enable them to make healthier dietary choices.

Stage-based Health Behavior Theories include:

- Transtheoretical Model (also called the Stages of Change Model) [42]
- Precaution-Adoption Process Model [43]
- Integrated Change (I-Change) Model [44, 45]
- Health Action Process Approach [46]
- Model of Action Phases [47]

Transtheoretical Model

The Transtheoretical Model, shown in Figure 2, is one of the most commonly used stage-based theories. It proposes that as people change a behavior, they move through these 5 stages [42].

I. Precontemplation. Precontemplators are not thinking about changing a behavior in the next 6 months. Some are not aware that they need to make a change. For instance, individuals who learn their blood lipid levels are too high during a check-up are unaware precontemplators—without blood test results, they do not know they need to eat less fat or get more exercise. Another example of unaware precontemplators are people who have been advised they have high blood lipids, but were not told that changes are needed to protect their health. A second group of precontemplators knows they need to change, but are not putting thought into why or how they might change. These unengaged contemplators may not realize or admit (deny) to themselves how serious their health condition is ("It's no big deal to have high blood lipids—lots of people do!"). They may

Figure 2. The Transtheoretical Model [40, 42]

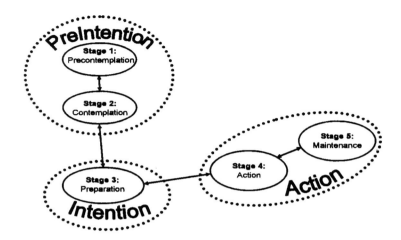

have other pressures that do not allow them to focus on changing ("My life is so hectic, I just can't think about it right now"). A third group of precontemplators are those who have tried to change but found it so difficult that they gave up. These beaten down precontemplators feel they have no alternative but to live with the problem and its health effects.

2. Contemplation. Contemplators are thinking about making a behavior change sometime soon—usually in the next 6 months. They spend time thinking, talking, and learning about their health behavior. Contemplators start identifying personal strengths and benefits and barriers to change, and weighing the advantages and disadvantages of continuing their current behavior or changing it. For contemplators, the perceived negatives of changing outweigh the positives. Common negatives include dislike of new foods (e.g., whole milk vs. 1% or non-fat, regular vs. diet soft drinks), monetary costs (e.g., buying exercise shoes), and time and effort costs (e.g., learning to read food labels, prepare food differently, or count carbohydrates). When the positives of health behavior changes (e.g., feeling better, being able to do the things they enjoy without getting out of breath or feeling pain, finding out they do enjoy the taste of new foods or that reading labels is easy) start to outweigh the negatives, contemplators begin making plans to change and move into the preparation stage. Some people are chronic contemplators—they spend a long time (maybe years) analyzing their problem and vowing they will change, but the right time to start changing never arrives.

3. *Preparation.* Preparers intend to change their behavior very soon—usually in the next month. They continue assessing themselves and their behavior and become progressively more confident that they will be able to make changes. The positives of changing now outweigh the negatives. Preparers commit to change, start to make a workable plan for overcoming the problem behavior, and may even begin taking small steps toward changing their behavior. For example, they might join a health club, consult a dietitian, buy a grill, or try reduced-calorie salad dressing. Changing a behavior takes a lot of willpower and energy. Preparers may experience disapproval of others who may be jealous, or feel threatened or inconvenienced by the change. Adequately preparing for change helps them to stay on track and avoid abandoning plans to change.

4. *Action.* Actors have taken steps to change their health behaviors within the past 6 months *and* have reached a level of behavior that experts believe will reduce disease risk. For example, most health experts believe Americans should eat 5 to 9 servings of fruits and vegetables daily. In this stage, **self-efficacy** (confidence that one will succeed) and perceptions about the benefits of changing increase. Actors make plans for coping with factors (e.g., motivation, people, situations) that may disrupt their progress. Some want help from friends, family, or professionals. To stay motivated, some give themselves small self-rewards (e.g., going to a movie, getting a manicure) for reaching a personal goal (e.g., eating 5 servings of fruits and vegetables every day for 2 weeks).

5. *Maintenance.* Maintainers have carried out the behavioral change (e.g., walking for 30 minutes daily) long enough (usually 6 months) that it has become part of their new lifestyle. The main goal of this stage is to continue to practice the changed behavior and avoid going back to their old habits. To prevent a return to previous behaviors, maintainers may think about how much progress they made [e.g., by keeping pictures of their heavier self on their bathroom mirror] and admit that there is a danger they could be tempted to revert to their old behavior.

Transtheoretical Model Stage Summary [42]

Stage 1—Precontemplation: not intending to change behavior in the next 6 months

Stage 2—Contemplation: intending to change behavior in the next 6 months

Stage 3—Preparation: intending to change behavior in the next month

Stage 4—Action: consistently changed behavior within the last 6 months

Stage 5—Maintenance: changed behavior for longer than the last 6 months

---

Precaution-Adoption Process Model [43]

The Precaution-Adoption Process Model shown in Figure 3 is another common stage-based behavior change theory. As you can see, it is very similar to the Transtheoretical Model. One difference is that the Transtheoretical Model specifies when individuals plan to make a change or how long they have maintained a change. A second difference is the Precaution-Adoption Process Model separates unaware and unengaged precontemplators into Stages 1 and 2. A third difference is the Precaution-Adoption Process Model recognizes that some may choose not to change. Those in Stage 4 may have decided they do not want to change, perhaps because they repeatedly tried and failed (beaten down precontemplators) or because they feel changing is too hard and the benefits of changing aren't worth it. Precaution-Adoption Process Model Stages 3, 5, 6, and 7 are comparable to the contemplation, preparation, action, and maintenance stages, respectively.

Figure 3. The Precaution-Adoption Process Model [40, 41, 43]

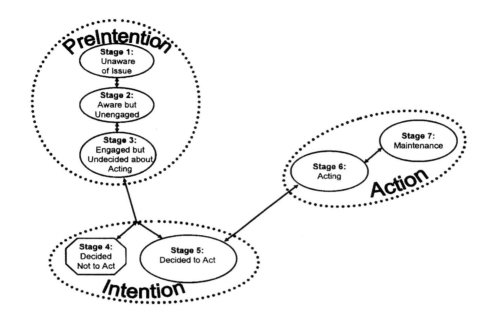

Moving Through the Stages

Moving through the stages may occur quickly, but it usually takes considerable time. People may stay in any one of the stages for a long time. Behavior change doesn't always progress forward, people often return to an earlier stage. For instance, a woman who was in the action stage for exercising 30 minutes daily may return to the preparation stage if she finds it too difficult to continue exercising when the weather gets cold. The number of people who have lost weight and regained it or stopped and restarted smoking illustrate that sliding back one or more stages is common. Some may move forward and backward through the stages several times before reaching maintenance. Even those who decided they do not want to modify their behavior may change their minds later on. Health professionals can help individuals learn from the past and try new approaches

[48]. For example, if winter weather derailed exercise plans, a new approach would be to find activities that can be done inside. For people who do not want to change right now, health professionals can be supportive by letting them know that help will be available when they are ready.

Put Your Knowledge Into Practice

Think about a behavior that you or someone you know well has wanted to change. Maybe this person wanted to start exercising regularly, drink fewer soft drinks, or eat more vegetables. What stage is this person in right now? (Try modifying Table 3 to assess the person's stage.) Did the person reach the maintenance stage? If so, how long did it take the person to reach the maintenance stage? Did the person revisit any of the previous stages after having moved to a later stage?

Table 3. Example of a Question that Can Help Determine
a Person's Stage of Change

Do you <u>eat 5 or more servings of fruits and vegetables</u> daily? *	Transtheoretical Model Stage	Precaution-Adoption Process Model Stage
A. No		
Why?		
1. *Because I don't know if my current diet is negatively affecting my health.*	Precontemplation	Stage 1: Unaware
2. *I know my current diet is negatively affecting my health, but I haven't thought about why or how I should change it.*	Precontemplation	Stage 2: Unengaged
3. *I just don't want to change my diet.*	Precontemplation	Stage 4: Decided not to act
4. *I don't practice this behavior right now, but I intend to start in the next 6 months.*	Contemplation	Stage 3: Aware but unengaged **
5. *I don't practice this behavior right now, but I intend to start in the next month.*	Preparation	Stage 5: Decided to act **
B. Yes		
How long have you been doing this?		
1. *Less than 6 months*	Action	Stage 6: Action **
2. *More than 6 months*	Maintenance	Stage 7: Maintenance **

*To adapt this for other behaviors, replace the underlined words with another behavior, such as drink 3 cups of milk, limit soft drink intake to 8 ounces or less, eat 4 servings of whole grains.

**Although the Precaution-Adoption Process Model does not specify a specific time for engaging in an activity, the time frames proposed by the Transtheoretical Model may be useful in determining when a behavior will be practiced or for how long a behavior has been practiced.

WHAT FACTORS INFLUENCE BEHAVIOR CHANGE AND MOVEMENT THROUGH THE STAGES OF CHANGE?

To help people move through the stages of change, it is important to consider the factors that influence behavior and promote behavior change. Research has revealed many factors are key influencers of health and dietary behaviors. These influencers are categorized into three levels or "spheres of influence": personal, social environment, and physical environment. The spheres and diet and health behaviors constantly interact with each other. The effect of these interactions is called **reciprocal determinism** (Figure 4).

Figure 4. Reciprocal Determinism is the constant interaction of people's behavior and the spheres of influence (Physical Environment, Social Environment, Personal) and the effects caused by these interactions [58. 59].

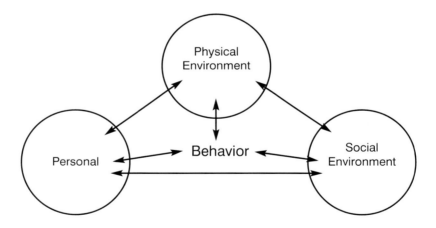

Let's look at key health and dietary behavior influencers in each sphere and how we might leverage them to create interventions that help consumers make healthier choices. These influencers, as you will see later in this chapter, were derived from the most commonly used decision-oriented health behavior theories. Stage-based theories explain *how* behavior changes and decision-oriented theories explain why a behavior is (or will be) practiced [49, 50].

Personal Sphere

The personal sphere factors are those that are within an individual, such as attitudes, knowledge, and self-confidence. Although they are within an individual, it is important to remember most factors can be altered by the person's behavior and the social and physical environment spheres. Key personal factors are described below.

Attitudes

Attitudes are one's beliefs, feelings, and values about a health condition (e.g., body weight) or behavior (e.g., eating less fat). Attitudes exert a strong influence on whether one decides or intends to change a behavior. Attitudes can be divided into three subgroups.

- **Salience of behavior** is a person's beliefs about how important it is to perform a behavior, such as not eating meat, losing weight, or taking nutrient supplements.

- **Experiential attitudes** are emotions about a health condition or behavior. A woman might have negative emotions (sad, angry, embarrassed) about being overweight or eating a special diet, but have positive emotions (happy, glad) about going to the gym.

- **Instrumental attitudes** are feelings that develop after evaluating the pros and cons of a health condition or behavior. For instance, the pros of being overweight and not dieting might be that the person can continue to eat as much as desired or not exercise at all. The cons might include being out of breath when walking to class or having a hard time fitting into classroom desks. The pros of losing weight could be feeling better and worrying less about health problems. The cons might be becoming stressed by going on a weight loss diet and fear of feeling hungry. The process of evaluating or weighing the pros and cons of a condition or behavior is called **decisional balance**.

Internal Resources

Internal resources are one's personal intellectual, psychological, and physical resources that can be used to achieve a goal, such as increasing lean body mass. Internal resources include the following.

- **Knowledge** is one's understanding of a health or nutrition problem and the value placed on taking a specific action, such as comprehending the risk of high blood lipid levels and the value of health behaviors (e.g., increasing fiber intake or exercising) that lower lipid levels. Knowledge is also affected by **health literacy**, which is "the degree to which individuals have the capacity to obtain, process, and understand basic health information and services needed to make appropriate health decisions" [51]. Knowledge is an important internal resource because research suggests that people with more nutrition knowledge tend to eat healthier diets than those who are less well informed [22].

- **Abilities and skills** are one's capability of making decisions about one's health and putting knowledge into action, such as meal planning or selecting lower fat items in a restaurant. Knowledge and abilities and skills develop through schooling, media exposure, and prior experience with things (e.g., food products, exercise equipment), activities (e.g., following special diets, joining support groups), institutions (e.g., health clubs, insurance companies), and/or individuals (e.g., health care professionals, coaches, teachers, friends, family) related to a health behavior.

- **Psychology** includes one's mental health status, mood, and personality characteristics. Positive emotions (e.g., joy, satisfaction, contentment) help build an individual's capacity to take actions that optimize health and well-being whereas mental disturbance or negative mood states (e.g., fear, anxiety, depression) diminish the capacity to protect one's health [52]. Personality characteristics, such as conscientiousness and agreeableness, may positively influence weight status and diet and exercise behaviors whereas impulsiveness may exert a negative influence [10, 53-56]. Resilience—or how people view life and use their resources (e.g., money, knowledge, skill, self-esteem, social support system) to bounce back from adversity and protect their health is another personality characteristic that supports health behavior change [57, 58].

- **Biology** includes factors that moderate the ability to take action on oneself or one's environment. Some factors generally cannot be altered (e.g., gender, life stage, genetic background) whereas others can be changed (e.g., physical health status, addictions, weathering). Gender and life stage can play a role in health and the outcomes of health behavior change in a variety of ways. For instance, men typically have more lean body mass, which usually allows them to lose weight faster than women. Premenopausal women tend to have higher HDL (good) cholesterol levels than men, even those who exercise regularly. Genetic predispositions, such as a family history of heart disease or longevity, can negatively or positively affect health. Having good physical health, being free of addictions, and not experiencing weathering (physical changes resulting from social adversity [59]) are internal biology resources that promote achievement of health goals.

- **Lifestyle** is a person's typical way of life, habits, and allocation of resources (e.g., time, energy, money, skills, knowledge) that reflect his or her values.

Personal Agency

Personal agency is a type of Internal Resource. It is one's perceived and actual ability to perform a behavior or exert power over a behavior and factors influencing the behavior, such as other people and the physical environment. Personal agency includes these aspects.

- **Perceived Control** is belief in one's ability to successfully control and manage oneself and one's environmental conditions so that it is possible to perform a particular behavior.

- **Self-Efficacy** is one's confidence in his or her ability to perform a specific behavior and effectively cope with temptations and consequences (such as eating fast food less often and coping with the increased effort to make meals at home and deal with complaints from other family members). When a group wants to bring about a change, their perceptions about their ability to perform the needed behaviors is called group efficacy or collective efficacy [60]. For example, a parent-teacher group may advocate a change in school policy to provide physical education for students. A community group may work to establish a local farmers' market to make fresh produce available to inner city residents.

- **Self-Regulation** is the ability to control one's behavior and emotions by using techniques like self-monitoring, self-appraisal, self-contracting, goal setting/planning, self-reward/reinforcement, self-instruction, enlisting social support, and restructuring the physical environment. Self-regulation examples include tracking calorie intake and evaluating it daily. Making a "contract" with oneself to walk 10,000 steps daily and rewarding oneself with an appointment for a pedicure after fulfilling the contract for a week. Self-instruction could be talking oneself through a situation (e.g., There are so many high fat foods at this party! I am going to position myself near the fresh vegetable tray so I can keep my calorie intake under control). Getting a friend to go for walks can provide the social support needed to continue to practice a behavior.

Restructuring the environment might be keeping fewer snack foods on hand at home or using hallways at work where there are no vending machines.

- **Coping Capacity** is the ability to identify coping strategies that are available and likely to support performance of a behavior. It also includes the skill of using coping strategies effectively to manage performance of the behavior and any psychological/emotional and environmental consequences of engaging in the behavior. For example, a college student may feel guilty after eating more than he planned. To actively and appropriately cope with this situation, he enlists support from friends who help him keep a positive mindset and get back on track to achieve his dietary goals.

Outcome Expectations

Outcome expectations are an individual's beliefs about a behavior and the beneficial (or detrimental) results that are likely to occur as a result of performing the behavior. It includes these components.

- **Severity Perceptions** are beliefs about how harshly a behavior is likely to affect physical, psychological, social, and/or economic well-being. A man who believes that eating a high fat diet is likely to cause severe health effects (heart attack, cancer) is more likely to lower his fat intake than someone who doesn't believe the risks are severe.

- **Susceptibility and Threat (Risk) Perception** is one's belief that he or she is vulnerable to a negative health condition (e.g., overweight, disease) because of performing (or not performing) a behavior. It also includes how important the consequences of performing the behavior are to the individual. An example is a woman who believes she is at risk for Type 2 diabetes because other family members have the condition. Because she feels vulnerable, she is more likely to change her behavior (e.g., lose weight, exercise more) than someone who isn't convinced he or she is vulnerable.

Social Norms

Social norms are written and unwritten rules that define "appropriate" thoughts, feelings, and behaviors of a culture and exert pressure on people to believe and behave in a certain way. Social norms include these facets.

- **Social Expectations** are beliefs about what important others (e.g., friends, families, colleagues) expect in one's behavior and one's motivation to comply with expectations. For instance, a social expectation in some families is to eat dinner together every day. Teens who wish to please their parents will try to comply with their parents' expectations.
- **Perceived Norms** are beliefs about how others behave. Perceptions about how others behave can be erroneous. For example, many college students mistakenly believe that most of their peers frequently consume large amounts of alcohol, when in reality only a small percent binge drink.

Put Your Knowledge Into Practice

Think about a health behavior that you need to change (e.g., eating more vegetables or whole grains, consuming less fat or salt, wearing a seatbelt, flossing your teeth daily, wearing sunscreen whenever you are in the sun more than a few minutes). Now, think about each of the personal factors above as they relate to your current behavior. What personal factors have kept you from changing your current behavior? What changes in your personal factors would help you adopt a new behavior?

Social Environment Sphere

The social environment sphere is external to an individual and includes interactions with other people, such as family, friends, colleagues, and institutions (e.g., educational, religious, political, and cultural groups). The social environment sphere can be altered by a person's behavior and the personal and physical environment spheres. Key social environment factors are described next.

- **Culture** is socially transmitted knowledge, behaviors, experience, beliefs, values, attitudes, meanings, hierarchies, and roles that distinguish members of one group from others. Culture also includes the degree to which one is acculturated to the prevailing culture. For instance, new immigrants' behaviors are likely to reflect values, beliefs, and practices from their country of origin whereas the values, beliefs, and practices of those who have lived in a new country for a long time tend be more like those of the new country. Food practices and preferences are often the last characteristics to change among immigrant groups. It is important to keep in mind that culture can be defined as ethnicity, race, and/or religion as well as social and personal networks.

- **Observational Learning** involves learning that occurs through exposure to other people and media [61, 62]. This learning can affect any of the personal sphere factors. For instance, a person's perceptions of the severity of a disease might change after observing the pain and suffering of a close relative who has cancer. On the other hand, seeing how easy it is for a friend to eat a delicious and low fat diet may alter one's self-efficacy with regard to eating a similar diet. The impact of observational learning seems to be especially important during the growing years. This is why health educators encourage parents to model health protective behaviors (e.g., eating a healthy diet, exercising, wearing seatbelts) and to watch television with children so they can help children draw accurate conclusions from what they see.

- **Social Support** includes psychological/emotional support, tangible aid and services (e.g., food stamps, counseling), information (advice, suggestions), and appraisals (constructive feedback for self-reevaluation). Social support may be provided by family and friends or by professionals, such as nutrition educators, legal aid advisors, religious leaders, and psychologists.

- **Social Equality** occurs when all people in a society have the same status and have equal legal rights (e.g., freedom of speech, right to vote) and equal access to education, health care, job opportunities, police and fire protection, and other social programs. Social inequalities (e.g., lack of affordable health insurance, prejudicial treatment) adversely affect physical and mental health and can present significant barriers to making health behavior changes.

- **Economic Environment** includes a person's overall purchasing power as a result of employment, income, expenses, cost of goods and services including taxes, and the strength and stability of the economic environment (e.g., recession). Purchasing power has a great impact on health because it can affect the type and amount of food a person can purchase, the quality (e.g., safety, size, location) of housing, availability of transportation, access to health care, and many other goods and services.

- **Political Environment** involves laws and regulations that affect (promote, restrict, modify) behaviors and options. Legislation requiring restaurant owners to post calories on menus may promote healthier food choices among patrons. Laws that restrict sales of alcohol to only those age 21 years and older limit access to this beverage. Taxing cigarettes or "junk food" at a high rate can modify behavior by causing people to purchase fewer of these items. School policies may dictate the types of foods that can be sold on campus before or after school.

Physical Environment Sphere

The physical environment sphere is the external surroundings and conditions in which one lives (i.e., natural and built environment) that affect behavior. The physical environment prompts individuals to act in certain ways. For instance, building a supermarket far from housing prompts people to drive instead of walking to the store. Physical surroundings and conditions can present **barriers** to changing health behaviors (e.g., unsafe neighborhoods prevent one from exercising after dark), provide **facilitators** to behavior change (e.g., the school gym opens in the evening for parents to exercise with their children), and offer **cues to action** (e.g., a reminder postcard from a health professional, a bowl of fruit on the table to prompt one to eat it as a snack). The physical environment sphere can be altered by a person's behavior and the personal and social environment spheres. Key physical environment factors affecting health are described next.

- **Information Environment** includes information availability and accessibility, information sources (e.g., health professionals vs. non-experts), media channels (e.g., television, Internet, advertising), information quality (accuracy, completeness, readability), and tone (positive, threatening) used to present the information.

- **Health Behavior Specific Environments** vary depending on the health behavior of interest. In the case of diet, the environment for this health behavior includes characteristics like food availability and accessibility in the home and community, feeding styles used by parents, mealtime rituals, body image norms, and nutrition information. In the case of exercise, the environment for this health behavior includes resources needed for exercise (e.g., equipment and space) and prevalence of resources that deter exercise (e.g., energy/time-saving conveniences). If smoking is the behavior of interest, its environment includes cigarette access (e.g., cost, ease of purchasing) and environments that support or deter the activity (e.g., smoke-free workplaces).

- **Technological Environment** involves factors affecting the development and distribution of technological advances, such as new products (e.g., medications, fat substitutes), new manufacturing methods (e.g., those that reduce cost or increase accessibility to a product), and new marketing and information dissemination methods (e.g., Internet). Access to technology frequently depends on the Economic Environment.

- **Health Care Environment** components are availability, quality, and accessibility of health care professionals, facilities, medications, and educational and social (e.g., WIC) programs that help individuals improve their health. The Health Care Environment is closely related to the Economic Environment.

Put Your Knowledge Into Practice

Think about a health behavior that you want to change. Now, think about each of the components of your social environment and physical environment as they relate to your current behavior. What social environment and physical environment factors support your current behavior and deter change? What changes could you make to your social environment and physical environment to help you implement a new behavior?

HOW ARE THE FACTORS
THAT AFFECT BEHAVIOR CHANGE RELATED?

As you now know, behaviors and the personal, social environment, physical environment spheres constantly interact and change each other (see Figure 4). Thus, changing one aspect of a behavior is likely to affect other behavioral aspects as well as all of the spheres. Many decision-oriented health behavior theories have been developed to describe why people behave the way they do and suggest why behavior change may occur. These theories can help health professionals identify the factors within each sphere (personal, social, environment) to address in health promotion interventions designed to change behaviors. This chapter discusses four of the most commonly used decision-oriented theories in health promotion and nutrition education.

- The Health Belief Model
- Theory of Reasoned Action, Theory of Planned Behavior, Integrated Behavioral Model
- The Social Cognitive Theory
- The Ecological Model

Health Belief Model [60, 63]

The Health Belief Model proposes that an individual's behavior is determined by the interactions between internal resources (e.g., age, gender, personality, knowledge), perceived threat (disease susceptibility and severity), outcome expectations (benefits), barriers, self-efficacy, and cues to action (see Figure 5). For example, if a man's parents both had heart disease, he may feel that he is very likely to develop heart disease (perceived susceptibility). If his parents died from heart disease complications, he might be even more concerned (perceived severity). If he had observed that his aunt who ate a healthy diet and exercised did not have heart disease complications, he may believe that those behaviors could really make a difference (perceived benefits). He may want to make changes, but he believes healthy foods cost too much and that he does not have time to

Figure 5. Health Belief Model [60, 63]

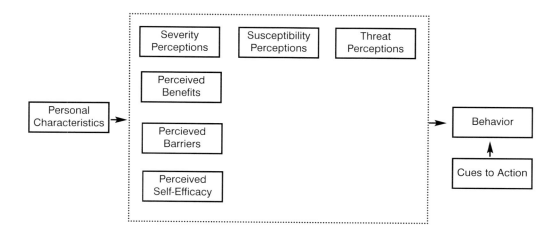

exercise (perceived barriers). If he believes he is able to make the changes (self-efficacy), he may be more likely to actually change behaviors than if he does not believe he is capable of performing the new behavior. Although he may be influenced by susceptibility, severity, benefits, barriers, and self-efficacy, he may not change his behavior until there is a cue to action, such as being diagnosed with high blood pressure.

THEORY OF REASONED ACTION, THEORY OF PLANNED BEHAVIOR, AND INTEGRATED BEHAVIORAL MODEL [64, 65]

The Theory of Reasoned Action was created first, then extended to become the Theory of Planned Behavior, and enhanced again to become the Integrated Behavioral Model (Figure 6). The Integrated Behavioral Model proposes that intention to perform a behavior is the result of interactions between attitudes, personal agency, and social norms, all of which can be affected by internal resources. It further proposes that actually performing a behavior is the result of intention to perform the behavior as well as attitudes toward the salience of the behavior, social and physical environment barriers, and internal resources of knowledge, skills, and habits. For example if a teen-age girl feels positively about eating fruits and vegetables (experiential attitude) and believes the pros of eating fruits and vegetables outweigh the cons (instrumental attitudes), she may have a very positive attitude toward eating fruits and vegetables. But, she may perceive that her friends don't eat fruits and vegetables (social norms) and that she will be considered very "uncool" if she eats fruit and vegetables (social expectations). She also may feel she has no control (perceived control) over the shopping and food preparation at home or the foods available at school or in the local corner-store. As you can see, all of these factors, attitudes, social norms, and personal agency interact to influence this teen's intention to eat fruits and vegetables.

Figure 6. Integrated Behavioral Model (An extension of the Theory of Reasoned Action and Theory of Reasoned Action and Theory of Planned Behavior) [64, 65]

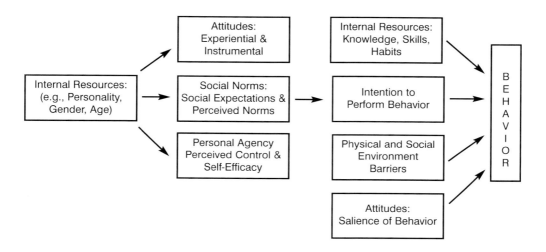

Intention to behave is a strong predictor of whether one will perform a behavior. Even if intention is strong, other factors influence whether a behavior will occur. Let's say the teen-age girl has a positive attitude toward eating fruits and vegetables, believes her friends eat these foods and want her to also eat them, and that her mother is willing to purchase more produce—all of these are supportive of eating more fruits and vegetables. If the family cannot afford to buy what is available at the grocery store (environment barrier), doesn't know how to prepare them (internal resource), or thinks eating these foods isn't very important (salience of behavior), it will be difficult to turn intentions into actual behavior.

Social Cognitive Theory [61, 62]

Social Cognitive Theory was originally called Social Learning Theory. Reciprocal determinism is a key premise of Social Cognitive Theory. That is, this theory proposes that people's behavior, personal characteristics, and social and physical environments constantly interact to influence each other (see Figure 4). This theory also proposes that people can restructure their environments to make it easier to perform a healthy behavior or not perform an unhealthy behavior (e.g., smoking, eating fried food often). This restructuring can be achieved by individuals or a group of people who work together toward a common goal. Other components of this theory include outcome expectations, self-regulation, self-efficacy, observational learning, group efficacy, and environmental facilitators (e.g., providing tools and resources that help people make behavior changes).

Ecological Models [66]

Ecology refers to the interaction between an organism and its environment. In the behavioral sciences, ecological models focus on how people interact with all aspects of their social and physical environments. Ecological models of health behavior propose that an individual's behaviors are the result of interactions between the personal, social environment, and physical environment spheres. According to these models, optimally effective behavior change programs address all spheres of influence.

Put Your Knowledge Into Practice

Take a close look at each of the decision-oriented theories described above. How are they similar? How are they different? How do you think they are related to stage-based theories?

What Is the Connection between Stage-Based and Decision-Oriented Theories?

A review of the last two sections may lead you to wonder whether stage-based and decision-oriented theories can work together and if so, how. A current challenge in the field of health behavior change is that commonly used theories do not integrate the *how* of stage-based with the *why* of decision-oriented models [40, 67]. Few efforts have been made to incorporate ideas from stage-based and decision-oriented theories [44, 68] despite the potential such a combination offers for advancing health behavior change and intervention development [68]. The Polytheoretical Framework in Figure 7 is one attempt to merge a stage-based theory with key constructs from decision-oriented models and provide a more holistic view of the multitude of factors affecting health behavior change.

By enhancing the Precaution Adoption Process Model, the Polytheoretical Framework describes both the how and why of behavior change and places change within in the context of multiple spheres of influence. The framework proposes that cues to action from the physical and social environments, observational learning, and internal resources help individuals become aware of and engaged with a health behavior issue so they can move through the three preintention stages. Internal resources, outcome expectations, attitudes, social norms, personal agency, and culture influence movement from Stage 3 to intention. It further proposes that personal agency, attitudes, and cues to action from the physical and social environments affect movement from Stage 5 to action.

There Are So Many Theories, Which One Should I Use?

Health behavior change theories only began to emerge in the 1940s, thus there is still a great deal we do not know about how people change behaviors. This isn't so surprising when you think about the wide array of health behaviors (e.g., eating, exercising, substance use, wearing seatbelts, brushing and flossing teeth, organ donations, sunscreen use, condom use, bike helmet use, preventive health practices such as immunizations and mammograms). Another factor to consider is the diversity of audiences—even if the audience is "women" think about how many different subgroups of women there are (e.g., college age vs. older women, new mothers vs. empty nest mothers, women who work outside the home vs. stay-at-home moms, healthy vs. ill women, health conscious vs. not health conscious women, limited resource vs. high income women). Each of these audiences has different needs, interests, knowledge, habits, values, motivations, and health challenges. If you multiply the number of health behaviors by the number of audiences, you can see why there might be so many different health behavior theories—*different researchers* have documented that *different* factors seem to affect *different* behaviors and *different* audiences differently and, as a result, have proposed *different* theories!

No one theory consistently outperforms others when it comes to predicting or explaining behavior [69-74]. Numerous studies also have not led to a consensus on which theory is most useful [75]. However, the interventions that most effectively help people make changes to improve their health are guided by health behavior theory and the target audience's personal, social environment, and physical environment spheres of influence. Mounting evidence indicates that certain constructs seem to be especially important in promoting change. Attitudes, personal agency, and social norms exert a strong influence on whether a person decides or intends to perform a health behavior. Moving from intention to action is most affected by personal agency, environment cues to action, self-regulation, and salience of the behavior itself.

Selecting the theory (or theories) most suitable for guiding the development of an intervention requires an understanding of: a) the constructs in each sphere of influence that frequently affect health behaviors, b) how commonly used theories apply constructs to explain behavior, c) the health problem that is the focus of an intervention, and d) the intervention target audience's needs, interests, values, motivations, attitudes, knowledge, and environment. This chapter provides the background needed to gain an understanding of a) and b). To gain an in-depth understanding of a health

Figure 7. The Polytheoretical Framework merges the stage-based Precaution-Adoption Process Model with key constructs from the most commonly used health behavior theories.

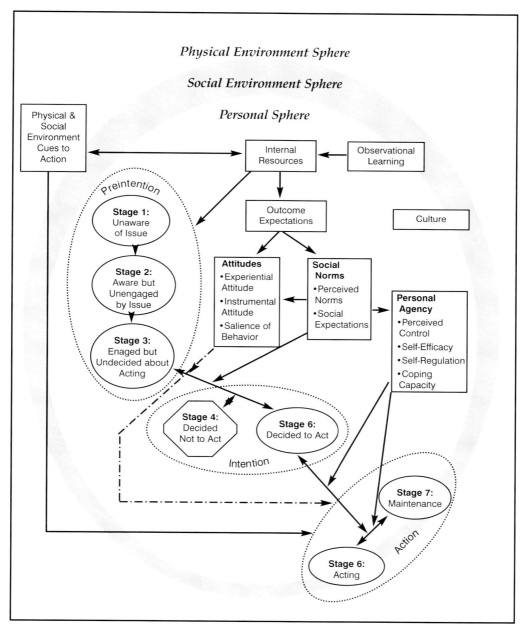

problem, examine reports about its prevalence, development, prevention, and treatment. Review reports of previous interventions and studies that dealt with the health problem and pay close attention to the suggestions for future research. To learn about the target audience, interview them to discover their core values and goals, observe their behaviors, visit areas where they live and take close notice of their physical environment, find out about their lifestyles and how they spend their time and money, and read reports describing their needs, lifestyle, and concerns. The more you know about your audience, the more likely you are to create interventions that are targeted and tailored specifically to them. Targeted and tailored interventions are personally relevant and meaningful to the audience, which increases the likelihood that the audience will pay attention to the intervention's health messages and, in turn, boosts the chances they will intend or actually perform a behavior [76].

Put Your Knowledge Into Practice

Think about a health behavior that many students on a local college campus need to change. Which constructs from the three spheres (i.e., personal, physical environment, and social environment) seem to influence the behavior? Which theory or theories do you think best explain why students do or do not engage in this behavior? What interventions have been used to change this behavior in similar communities? What are the students' needs, interests, values, motivations, attitudes, knowledge, and environment related to the behavior?

HOW CAN I MAXIMIZE THE CHANCES MY INTERVENTION WILL BE TARGETED AND TAILORED TO MY AUDIENCE?

The PRECEDE-PROCEED Planning Model can help health promotion experts apply health behavior theories and design interventions that are effective and readily accepted by the target audience [77, 78]. The PRECEDE component of the model was developed in response to the idea that a "diagnosis" of the problem is needed before an intervention plan is made. PRECEDE stands for Predisposing, Reinforcing, and Enabling Constructs in

Educational/Environmental Diagnosis and Evaluation. The PROCEED component addresses the influence of environmental factors on health behaviors and outcomes. PROCEED stands for Policy, Regulatory, and Organizational Constructs in Educational and Environmental Development.

This model is composed of the 8 steps described below (Table 4) [78, Note 1]. According to the model, during each step it is important to get input from the target audience, set priorities by selecting goals that are the most important and changeable, and set measurable objectives. A measurable goal describes who will do what, how much, and when. For example, the intervention participant will eat five servings of fruits and vegetables each day after completing the first three lessons.

Table 4. Summary of the PRECEDE-PROCEED Steps

Step 1 Social Assessment
Step 2 Epidemiological, Behavioral, and Environmental Assessment
Step 3 Educational and Ecological Phase
Step 4 Administrative and Policy Assessment and Intervention Alignment
Step 5 Intervention Implementation
Step 6 Process Evaluation
Step 7 Impact Evaluation
Step 8 Outcome Evaluation

Step 1 is social assessment. During this step, health promotion experts get to know the community by interviewing, observing, and surveying them. The goal is to understand the community's perceived needs, interests, resources, and readiness to change. Another goal is to develop partnerships with the community and get them interested in and supportive of the future intervention. "Community" is defined as a group who shares similar interests, beliefs, values, and norms. They may be a virtual (e.g., Internet bloggers) or actual community (e.g., college campus).

Step 2 is the epidemiological, behavioral, and environmental assessment phase. The focus of the epidemiological assessment is to identify the health problems of the community, determine behavioral and environmental factors that affect the health problems, and set priorities by developing measurable objectives for the intervention program addressing the health problems. The behavioral assessment's purpose is to gain an understanding of behaviors that contribute to the health problem and the effect of the problem on quality of life. These include behaviors of the individual with the health problem, people who directly affect the individual, and policy makers who affect the individual's social and physical environment. For example, teens often do not drink enough milk. The behaviors of their parents (e.g., not buying milk) and policy makers at school (e.g., only selling whole milk at lunch) may directly affect the teen's milk intake. The environmental evaluation examines factors in the social and physical environment that affect a health behavior. Knowing which of these factors could be modified (e.g., selling low fat or flavored milk at school) helps focus intervention priorities and objectives.

Step 3 is the educational and ecological phase. During this phase, intervention planners use behavioral and environment assessment information from Step 2 to determine the factors that need to occur before a behavior changes (Predisposing and Enabling factors) and those that will reward and reinforce the new behavior (Reinforcing and Enabling factors). Predisposing factors include internal resources and self-efficacy. Reinforcing factors include self-reward and social support. Enabling factors include social and physical environments that support initiation and continuation of the behavior.

Step 4 is administrative and policy assessment and intervention alignment. During this phase, the intervention planner selects the intervention components and aligns (matches) them with the priorities identified in Step 2. Next, the planner determines the resources, policies, barriers, and facilitators that will be needed to implement and sustain the intervention.

The change processes construct from the Transtheoretical Model can be useful in designing intervention components during Steps 3 and 4. Change processes (Table 5) are the activities that can help people move through the stages of change [79] They can be put into two broad groups: experiential and behavioral. Experiential change processes involve changing the way people think and feel about their behavior—they relate to their basic personal reasons for behaving (e.g., eating) the way they do and changing. They are used mostly during the preintention phase [79]. Behavioral processes involve actually changing behavior and are used mostly in the intention and action stages.

Step 5 is the implementation of the intervention. *Step 6* focuses on process evaluation (assessment of whether the intervention was implemented as it was planned). *Step 7* is impact evaluation (assessment of changes in predisposing, reinforcing, enabling, behavioral, and environmental factors). *Step 8* is outcome evaluation (measurement of the interventions' effect on health and quality of life). The Logic Model can help the intervention planner put the PRECEDE-PROCEED Model in action.

Table 5. Change Processes from the Transtheoretical Model

Experiential Change Processes
Consciousness raising involves increasing awareness of the causes, consequences, and treatments for a particular problem health behavior. Examples are reading an article, attending a class, seeing a doctor, and visiting a website.
Social liberation focuses on creating and/or using alternatives that are supportive of behavior change efforts. Examples include using nutrition facts labels to make food selections and ordering heart healthy entrees featured on restaurant menus.
Dramatic relief is an emotionally arousing experience that causes a strong emotional reaction to the potential consequences of a problem health behavior. Examples include real-life tragedies, personal testimonials, and graphic movies.
Self re-evaluation occurs when people imagine themselves with and without the problem behavior. It helps them see how their problem health behaviors conflict with their self-image and values and assess the costs (time, energy, stress) associated with the problem. Examples include visualizing themselves without the problem behavior and self-assessment checklists.

Environmental re-evaluation is considering how one's behaviors affect the people around them. Examples include empathy training and documentaries.

Behavioral Change Processes

Commitment (self-liberation) is an individual's belief that he or she can make changes and commit to making those changes. Examples include making a self-contract or New Year's Resolution and telling friends about the planned change.

Counter conditioning is learning new healthy strategies that can be used to replace previous unhealthy lifestyles or strategies. Examples include learning to refocus energy on another task such as surfing the Internet or texting a friend instead of binge eating, learning relaxation techniques to prevent stress driven eating, or making substitutes like having a small order of fries instead of a large one.

Stimulus control involves modifying the environment to remove temptations and elements that trigger the problem behavior and sabotage efforts for change. An example is identifying temptations in one's environment (e.g., too many snack foods on hand) and making plans for avoiding them (e.g., buying lower calorie snack foods or fewer snack foods).

Reinforcement management is positive reinforcements (rewards like compliments, special privileges, and gifts) that support and reinforce behavior change. Examples include positive self-talk, giving oneself "permission" to take time for a long bath, and rewarding oneself with small gifts after reaching a goal.

Helping relationships involve people who provide the social support needed to help an individual make a behavior change. Examples include joining a support group, finding a buddy, and developing a relationship with a health care provider.

The Logic Model

The Logic Model is a tool for planning, implementing, managing, and evaluating health and nutrition intervention programs. It shows what is needed (investments) and must be done (activities) to achieve the goals of a program (e.g., increase intake of whole grains).

The Logic Model has six basic components: situation (identifying a health behavior problem that needs an intervention program), inputs (resources such as time, money), outputs (activities conducted or products created that reach targeted participants), outcomes (results that occur from delivering outputs), assumptions (beliefs), and external factors that affect the program. Figure 8 shows a simple way to think about the components. You get very hungry because you skipped breakfast (situation). You believe apples taste good (assumption) and know they are available where you usually eat (external factor). So, you decide to buy an apple in the dining hall (inputs) and eat it (outputs), which makes you feel satiated

Figure 8. An Everyday Example of the Logic Model*

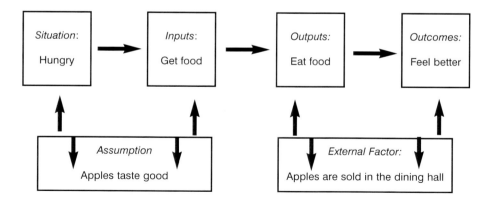

*Adapted from University of Wisconsin-Extension Program Development and Evaluation.
http://www.uwex.edu/ces/pdande/evaluation/powerpt/mguideslides.ppt#385.15.Everyday%20example

and happy (outcomes). Let's take a closer look at these components in more detail (see Figure 9).

Figure 9. Components of the Logic Model*

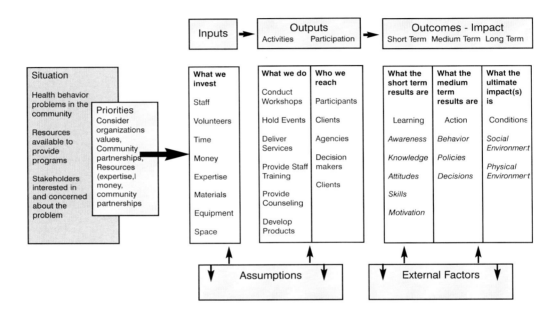

*Adapted from University of Wisconsin-Extension Program Development and Evaluation. http://www.uwex.edu/ces/pdande/evaluation/powerpt/mguideslides. ppt#385.15.Everyday%20example

Situation includes the health behavior problems in a community that need to be addressed in an intervention program and resources available to provide programs. Describing the situation requires investigating *why* the problem exists, *who* has the problem, *who* is interested in and concerned about the problem (stakeholders), and *what* can be changed to address the health behavior problem. There are usually more health behavior problems than can be addressed with the resources available.

Thus, once the situation is completely described and analyzed, it is time to set priorities. The criteria used to set priorities may be based on the goals and values of the organization that will offer an intervention program, as well as its resources (e.g., expertise, community partnerships, money), what others are doing in relation to the problem, and the goals, values, and interests of the target audience (i.e., those who will participate in the program). The target audience may be individuals with the health behavior problem, agencies that work with these individuals, or others. Those who set the priorities may include the organization that will provide the program, funders of the organization (e.g., philanthropic groups, government organizations), and the target audience. The programs that most successfully change behaviors usually include program participants in decision-making processes. Data collected during Step 1 (social assessment) and Step 2 (epidemiological, behavioral, and environmental assessment) of the PRECEDE-PROCEED Model provide much of the information needed to describe the situation component of the Logic Model.

Inputs are resources invested to reach desired outputs and outcomes. Inputs can include staff, volunteers, time, money, expertise, materials, equipment, and space for conducting the program (e.g., office and classroom space). **Outputs** are the activities (e.g., workshops, events, services, staff training, counseling) and products (e.g., posters, videos, blogs, podcasts) developed to address the priorities and reach the target audience. Activities and products lead to outcomes. **Assumptions** are beliefs that program planners have about the health problem or situation, priorities, inputs, outputs, expected outcomes, the target audience and how they may be affected by the program, and the effect of external factors on program success. Activities completed in Step 3 (educational and ecological phase) and Step 4 (administrative and policy assessment and intervention alignment) of the PRECEDE-PROCEED Model provide useful information about inputs, outputs, and assumptions.

Outcomes are the final goal. They are the changes that occur in the target audience and describe the effect the program has on the health behavior problem. *Short-term outcomes* are changes in the target audience's internal resources (e.g., increased awareness, knowledge, attitudes, skills, motivations). For example, a program may help parents become more aware of the health benefits of exercising and learn safe exercise techniques (skills). *Medium-term outcomes* are changes in the target audience's behavior (e.g., they may perform a behavior, set a policy, make a decision). Four months after attending the program, the parents have started walking their children to school every day instead of driving them. *Long-term outcomes* are changes in the social environment and physical environment. These may take years to achieve. The local park commission may add more sidewalks and bike paths around town to encourage more children to walk or bike to school and increase their physical activity. External factors are conditions in the social and physical environment that interact with and influence program outcomes as well as factors in the target audience's personal sphere (e.g., participants' attitudes, abilities and skills) that affect how they respond to the program. Step 7 (impact evaluation) and Step 8 (outcome evaluation) in the PRECEDE-PROCEED Model are analogous to the outcomes component of the Logic Model.

Why Use a Logic Model?

The Logic Model is a useful tool because, like a road map, it graphically shows where you are and what you'll need to get to where you want to be. That is, it helps to ensure that Step 5 (intervention implementation) and Step 6 (process evaluation) in the PRECEDE-PROCEED Model occur as planned. It can be used with programs of all sizes, ranging from large, long-term multi-part programs (e.g., health promotion programs for military families around the world) to small, short-term programs (e.g., a local community's 6-week 'shapeup' campaign or a health department's half-day health fair).

Developing a logic model when planning a program helps you know that key components have been considered. It also makes it easier to clearly explain to others (e.g., funders, program participants, program staff) how the program will work and what it will achieve. Once the program is underway, the Logic Model helps keep the program on track and helps program planners monitor the program and determine whether the program is likely to succeed. By keeping the program's Logic Model up to date and sharing it with project staff, everyone will know how the project is progressing and understand how they can help make the program a success. This model also is useful when reporting the program outcomes because it helps remind report writers to include short-, medium-, and long-term outcomes. To learn more about the Logic Model, visit http://www.uwex.edu/ces/pdande/evaluation/.

Put Your Knowledge Into Practice

Think once again about a health behavior that many students on a local college campus need to change. Use Figure 10 to create a Logic Model for a program that could help students change the problem behavior. Describe the situation. What do you think the priorities should be? What will you need to invest to create a program (inputs)? What activities will you do and who will you reach (outputs)? What assumptions are you making? What external factors from the target audience's personal sphere of influence as well as the social and physical environment likely affect the program? What are the desired short-, medium-, and long-term outcomes?

Figure 10. Put your knowledge into practice by completing this Logic Model

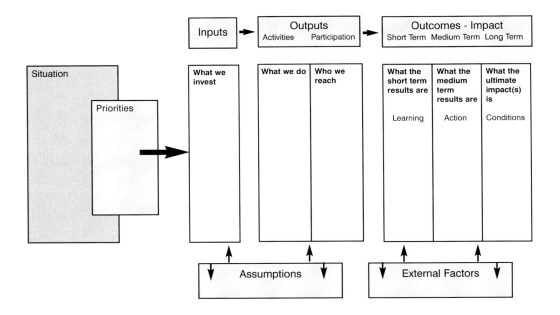

Notes

Note 1: Text in this section adapted from [80].

References

1. Glanz, K., et al., *Why Americans eat what they do: taste, nutrition, cost, convenience, and weight control concerns as influences on food consumption.* Journal of the American Dietetic Association, 1998. 98(10): p. 1118-26.

2. Neumark-Sztainer, D., et al., *Factors influencing food choices of adolescents: Findings from focus-group discussions with adolescents.* Journal of the American Dietetic Association, 1999. 99: p. 929-937.

3. Rappaport, L., et al., *Gender and age differences in food cognition.* Appetite, 1993. 20: p. 33-52.

4. Sporny, L. and I. Contento, *Stage of change in dietary fat reduction: Social psychological correlates.* Journal of Nutrition Education, 1995. 27(191-199).

5. Stewart, B. and A. Tinsley, *Importance of food choice influences for working young adults.* Journal of the American Dietetic Association, 1995. 95: p. 227-230.

6. Tuorila, H. and R. Pangborn, *Prediction of reported consumption of selected fat-containing foods.* Appetite, 1988. 11: p. 81-95.

7. Wilson, J., et al., *Data Tables: Combining results from USDA's 1994 and 1995 Continuing Survey of Food Intakes by Individuals and 1994 and 1995 Diet and Health Knowledge Survey, Table Set 5.* 1997, United States Department of Agriculture: Washington, DC.

8. Wirfalt, A. and R. Jeffery, *Using cluster analysis to examine dietary patterns: Nutrient intakes, gender, and weight status differ across food pattern clusters.* Journal of the American Dietetic Association, 1997. 97: p. 272-279.

9. Betts, N., et al., *What young adults say about factors affecting their food intake.* Ecology of Food and Nutrition, 1995. 34: p. 59-64.

10. Horacek, T. and N. Betts, *Students cluster into 4 groups according to the factors influencing their dietary intake.* Journal of the American Dietetic Association, 1998. 98: p. 1464-1467.

11. Rappoport, L., et al., Reasons for eating: An exploratory cognitive analysis. Ecology of Food and Nutrition, 1992. 28: p. 171-189.

12. Hayes, D. and C. Ross, *Concern with appearance, health beliefs, and eating habits.* Journal of Health and Social Behavior, 1987. 28: p. 120-130.

13. Mooney, K. and L. Walbourn, *When college students reject food: Not just a matter of taste.* Appetite, 2000. 36: p. 41-50.

14. Armstrong, J., E. Lange, and D. Stem, *Convenience as a factor in meal preparation among health-conscious adults.* Home Economics Research Journal, 1991. 19: p. 224-232.

15. Sloan, A.E., *What, when, and where America eats.* Food Technology, 2006. 60: p. 19-27.

16. Byrd-Bredbenner, C., *Food Preparation Knowledge and Attitudes of Young Adults: Implications for Nutrition Practice.* Topics in Clinical Nutrition, 2004. 19: p. 154-163.

17. Byrd-Bredbenner, C., *Food Preparation Knowledge and Confidence of Young Adults. Journal of Nutrition in Recipe & Menu Development*, 2005. 3: p. 37-50.

18. Sloan, E., *Demographic directions: Mixing up the market.* Food Technology, 2005. 59: p. 34-45.

19. Healy, M., *Ease trumps health in meal choices*, in USA Today. 2006: Washington, DC. p. 8D.

20. Axelson, M., T. Federline, and D. Brinberg, *A meta-analysis of food- and nutrition-related research.* Journal of Nutrition Education, 1985. 17: p. 51-54.

21. Crites, S. and S. Aikman, *Impact of nutrition knowledge on food evaluations.* European Journal of Clinical Nutrition, 2005. 59: p. 1191-1200.

22. Wardle, J., K. Parmenter, and J. Wller, *Nutrition knowledge and food intake.* Appetite, 2000. 34: p. 269-275.

23. McGinnis, J., J. Gootman, and V. Kraak, eds. *Food Marketing to Children and Youth: Threat or Opportunity?* 2006, National Academies Press: Washington, DC.

24. Byrd-Bredbenner, C., M. Finckenor, and A. Grenci, *A Television Program Affects Children's Nutrition Knowledge and Beliefs.* Journal of the American Dietetic Association, 2004. 104: p. A51.

25. Signorielli, N. and M. Lears, *Television and children's conceptions of nutrition: Unhealthy messages.* Health Communications, 1992. 4(4): p. 245-257.

26. Wiman, A. and L. Newman, *Television advertising exposure and children's nutritional awareness.* Journal of the Academy of Marketing Science, 1989. 17(2): p. 179-188.

27. Borzekowski, D. and T. Robinson, *The 30-second effect: An experiment revealing the impact of television commercials on food preferences of preschoolers.* Journal of the American Dietetic Association, 2001. 101(1): p. 42-46.

28. Galst, J. and M. White, *The unhealthy persuader: The reinforcing value of television and children's purchase-influence attempts at the supermarket.* Child Development, 1976. 47: p. 1089-1094.

29. Gorn, G.J. and M. Goldberg, *Behavioral evidence of the effects of televised food messages on children.* Journal of Consumer Research, 1982. 9: p. 200-205.

30. Taras, H., et al., *Television advertising and classes of food products consumed in a paediatric population.* International Journal of Advertising, 2000. 19: p. 487-493.

31. Boynton-Jarrett, R., et al., *Impact of television viewing patterns on fruit and vegetable consumption among adolescents.* Pediatrics, 2003. 112(6): p. 1321-1326.

32. Giammattei, J., et al., *Television watching and soft drink consumption: associations with obesity in 11- to 13-year old schoolchildren.* Archives of Pediatrics & Adolescent Medicine, 2003. 157: p. 882-886.

33. Halford, J., et al., *The effect of television (TV) food advertisements / commercials on food consumption in children.* Appetite, 2004. 42: p. 221-225.

34. Lindeman, M. and M. Vaananen, *Measurement of ethical food choice motives.* Appetite, 2000. 34: p. 55-59.

35. Martins, Y. and P. Pliner, *The development of the food motivation scale.* Appetite, 1998. 30: p. 94.

36. Rozin, P., *Towards a psychology of food and eating: From motivation to module to model to marker, morality, meaning and metaphor.* Current Directions In Psychological Science, 1996(5): p. 18-24.

37. Solheim, R. and H. Lawless, *Consumer purchase probability affected by attitude towards low-fat foods, liking, private body consciousness and information on fat and price.* Food Quality and Preference, 1996. 7: p. 137-143.

38. Steptoe, A. and T. Pollard, *Development of a measure of the motives underlying the selection of food: The Food Choice Questionnaire. Appetite, 1995. 25: p. 267-284.*

39. Glanz, K., B. Rimer, and K. Viswanath, eds. *Theory, research, and practice in health behavior and health education.* 4 ed. Health Behavior and Health Educ. Theory, Research, and Practice, ed. K. Glanz, B. Rimer, and K. Viswanath. 2008, Jossey-Bass: San Francisco.

40. Schuz, B., et al., *Predicting transitions from preintentional, intentional and actional stages of change.* Health Education Research, 2009. 24: p. 64-75.

41. Weinstein, N., A. Rothman, and S. Sutton, *Stage Theories of Health Behavior: Conceptual and Methodological Issues.* Health Psychology, 1998. 17: p. 290-299.

42. Prochaska, J., C. Redding, and K. Evers, eds. *The transtheoretical model and stages of change.* 4 ed. Health Behavior and Health Educ. Theory, Research, and Practice, ed. K. Glanz, B. Rimer, and K. Viswanath. 2008, Jossey-Bass: San Francisco.

43. Weinstein, N., P. Sandman, and S. Blalock, eds. *The precaution adoption process model.* 4 ed. Health Behavior and Health Educ. Theory, Research, and Practice, ed. K. Glanz, B. Rimer, and K. Viswanath. 2008, Jossey-Bass: San Francisco.

44. deVries, H., et al., *The general public's information needs and perceptions regarding hereditary cancer: an application of the Integrated Change Model.* Patient Education and Counseling, 2005. 56: p. 154-165.

45. Smeets, T., et al., *Effects of Tailored Feedback on Multiple Health Behaviors.* Annals of Behavioral Medicine, 2007. 33: p. 117–123.

46. Schwartzer, R., *Social-Cognitive Factors in Changing Health-Related Behaviors.* Current Directions in Psychological Science, 2001. 10: p. 47-51.

47. Gollwitzer, P., *Volitional Benefits of Planning,* in *The psychology of action,* P. Gollwitzer and J. Bargh, Editors. 1996, Guilford Press: New York. p. 287-312.

48. Sandoval, W., et al., *Stages of change: A model for nutrition counseling.* Topics in Clinical Nutrition, 1994. 9: p. 64-69.

49. Noar, S., M. Chabot, and R. Zimmerman, *Applying health behavior theory to multiple behavior change: Considerations and approaches.* Preventive Medicine, 2008. 46: p. 275-280.

50. Rimer, B., ed. *Models of individual health behaviors. 4 ed. Health Behavior and Health Education.* Theory, Research, and Practice, ed. K. Glanz, B. Rimer, and K. Viswanath. 2008, Jossey-Bass: San Francisco.

51. U.S. Department of Health and Human Services, *Health Communication, in Healthy People 2010, Understanding and Improving Health.* 2000, U.S. Government Printing Office: Washington, DC.

52. Fredrickson, B., Cultivating *Positive Emotions to Optimize Health and Well-Being. Prevention & Treatment,* 2000 3: p. Article 0001a.

53. Courneya, K.S. and L.M. Hellsten, *Personality correlates of exercise behavior, motives, barriers, and preferences: An application of the five-factor model.* Personality and Individual Differences, 1998. 24: p. 625-633.

54. Terracciano, A., et al., *Facets of Personality Linked to Underweight and Overweight.* Psychosomatic Medicine, 2009. 71(6): p. 682-689.

55. Brummett, B.H., et al., *Personality as a predictor of dietary quality in spouses during midlife.* Behavioral Medicine, 2008. 34(1): p. 5-10.

56. de Bruijn, G.-J., et al., *Is personality related to fruit and vegetable intake and physical activity in adolescents?* Health Education Research, 2005. 20(6): p. 635-644.

57. Almedom, A. and D. Glandon, *Resilience is not the absence of PTSD any more than health is the absence of disease.* J Loss and Trauma, 2007. 12: p. 127-143.

58. Antonovsky, A. and T. Sourani, *Family sense of coherence and family adaptation.* Journal of Marriage and Family Therapy, 1988. 50: p. 79-92.

59. Geronimus, A.T., *Understanding and Eliminating Racial Inequalities in Women's Health in the United States: The Role of the Weathering Conceptual Framework*. Journal of the American Medical Women's Association, 2001. 56: p. 133-136.

60. Champion, V. and C. Skinner, *The Health Belief Model, in Health Behavior and Health Education. Theory, Research, and Practice*, K. Glanz, B. Rimer, and K. Viswanath, Editors. 2008, Jossey-Bass: San Francisco.

61. Bandura, A., *Social Learning Theory*. 1977, Englewood Cliffs, NJ: Prentice-Hall.

62. Bandura, A., *Health promotion by social cognitive means*. Health Education and Behavior, 2004. 31: p. 143-164.

63. Becker, H., *The Health Belief Model and personal health behavior*. Health Education Monographs, 1974. 2: p. 324-473.

64. Ajzen, I., *The theory of planned behavior*. Organizational behavior and human decision processes, 1991. 50: p. 179-211.

65. Montano, D. and D. Kasprzyk, *Theory of reasoned action, theory of planned behavior, and the integrated behavioral model, in Health Behavior and Health Education. Theory, Research, and Practice*, K. Glanz, B. Rimer, and K. Viswanath, Editors. 2008, Jossey-Bass: San Francisco.

66. Sallis, J., N. Owen, and E. Fisher, eds. *Ecological Models of Health Behavior*. 4 ed. Health Behavior and Health Educ. Theory, Research, and Practice, ed. K. Glanz, B. Rimer, and K. Viswanath. 2008, Jossey-Bass: San Francisco.

67. Noar, S., *A health educator's guide to theories of health behavior*. Policy, Theory, and Social Issues, 2005-2006. 24: p. 75-92.

68. Lippke, S. and R. Plotnikoff, *The protection motivation theory within the stages of the transtheoretical model - Stage-specific interplay of variables and prediction of exercise stage transitions*. British Journal of Human Psychology, 2009. 14: p. 211-229.

69. Baranowski, T., K. Cullen, and J. Baranowski, *Psychosocial Correlates of Dietary Intake: Advancing Dietary Intervention*. Annual Review of Nutrition, 1999. 19: p. 17-40.

70. Baranowski, T., et al., *Are current health behavioral change models helpful in guiding prevention of weight gain efforts?* Obesity Research, 2003. 11: p. 23S-43S.

71. Brug, J., *Order is needed to promote linear or quantum changes in nutrition and physical activity behaviors: A reaction to 'A chaotic view of behavior change' by Resnicow and Vaughan*. International Journal of Behavioral Nutrition and Physical Activity, 2006. 3: p. 29-32.

72. Resnicow, K. and R. Vaughan, *A chaotic view of behavior change: A quantum leap for health promotion*. International Journal of Behavioral Nutrition and Physical Activity, 2006. 3: p. 25-30.

73. Rothman, A., *"Is there nothing more practical than a good theory?": Why innovations and advances in health behavior change will arise if interventions are used to test and refine theory.* International Journal of Behavioral Nutrition and Physical Activity, 2004. 1: p. 11-17.

74. Cerin, E., A. Barnett, and T. Baranowski, *Testing theories of dietary behavior change in youth using the mediating variable model with intervention programs.* Journal of Nutrition Education and Behavior, 2009. 41: p. 309-318.

75. Maddux, J., *Social cognitive models of health and exercise behavior: an introduction and review of conceptual issues.* Journal of Applied Sports Psychology, 1993. 5: p. 116-140.

76. Petty, R. and D. Wegener, *The Elaboration Likelihood Model: Current Status and Controversies, in Dual Process Theories in Social Psychology*, S. Chaiken and Y. Trope, Editors. 1999, Guilford Press: New York. p. 41–72.

77. Gielen, A., et al., eds. *Using the PRECEDE-PROCEED Model to Apply Health Behavior Theories.* 4 ed. Health Behavior and Health Education. Theory, Research, and Practice, ed. K. Glanz, B. Rimer, and K. Viswanath. 2008, Jossey-Bass: San Francisco.

78. Green, L. and M. Kreuter, *Health promotion planning: An educational and ecological approach.* 4th ed. 2005, New York: McGraw-Hill.

79. Cancer Prevention Research Center and University of Rhode Island. Detailed *Overview of the Transtheoretical Model.* undated [cited; Available from: http://www.uri.edu/research/cprc/TTM/detailedoverview.htm.

80. Byrd-Bredbenner, C. and M. Finckenor, Putting *The Transtheoretical Model Into Practice With Type 2 Diabetes Mellitus Patients.* Topics in Clinical Nutrition, 2000. 15: p. 44-58.

References

ABC News, October 21, 2009. Accessed on 11/14/2009 from: http://abcnews.go.com/Politics/Health/fda-scrutinizes-food-labels-cereals-smart-choices-program/story?id=8878025.

Abraido-Lanza, A. (2004). Immigrant Populations and Health. *Encyclopedia of Health & Behavior*, **2**. N. B. Anderson. Thousand Oaks/London/New Delhi, Sage Publications: 533-37.

Abraido-Lanza, A. et al. (2005). "Do healthy behaviors decline with greater acculturation? Implications for the Latino mortality paradox." *Social Science Medicine* **61**(6): 1243-55.

Adams, L. (1997). An overview of adolescent eating behavior barriers to implementing dietary guidelines. *Ann NY Acad Sci* **817**:36-48.

Ainsworth, B. et al. (2003). Personal, social, and physical environmental correlates of physical activity in African-American women in South Carolina. *Am J Prev Med* **25**:23-29S.

Albarran, N. et al. (2006). Dietary Behavior and type 2 diabetes care. *Patient Education and Counseling* **61**(2): 191-199.

Ajani, U. et al. (2004). "Body mass index and mortality among US male physicians." *Ann Epidemiol* **14**(10): 731-9.

Ajzen, I. (1991). "The theory of planned behavior." *Organizational behavior and human decision processes* **50**: 179-211.

al-Asfoor, D. et al. (1999). "Body fat distribution and the risk of noninsulin-dependent diabetes mellitus in the Omani population." *East Mediterr Health J* **5**(1): 14-20.

Albarran, N. et al. (2005). "Dietary behavior and type 2 diabetes care." *Patient Educ Couns.* **61**(2):191-199.

Almedom, A. and Glandon, D. (2007). "Resilience is not the absence of PTSD any more than health is the absence of disease." *J Loss and Trauma* **12**: 127-143.

American Academy of Pediatrics (2005). "Policy Statement: Breastfeeding and the use of human milk." **115** (2): 496-506.

American Heart Association. Heart, Healthy Grocery Shopping Made Simple. Accessed on 11/4/09, from http://www.americanheart.org/presenter.jhtml?identifier=2115

Andreyeva, T. et al. (2008). "Changes in perceived weight discrimination among Americans, 1995-1996 through 2004-2006." *Obesity (Silver Spring)* **16**(5): 1129-34.

Andrieu, E. et al. (2006). Low-cost diets: more energy, fewer nutrients. *Eur J Clin Nutr* **60**:434-436.

Antonovsky, A. and Sourani, T. (1988). "Family sense of coherence and family adaptation." *Journal of Marriage and Family Therapy* **50**:79-92.

Aquilino, W. (1997). "From adolescent to young adult: A prospective study of parent child relations during the transition to adulthood." *Journal of Marriage and the Family* **59**: 670-686.

Arimond, M. and Ruel, M. (2004). "Dietary diversity is associated with child nutritional status: evidence from 11 Demographic and Health Surveys." *J Nutr.* **134**(10): 2579-2585.

Arnett, J. (1997). Young people's conception of the transition to adulthood. *Youth and Society* **29**:3-21.

Arnett, J. (1998). Learning to stand alone: the contemporary American transition to adulthood in cultural and historical context. *Hum Dev* **41**:295-315.

Arnett, J. (1999). "Winston's "No Additives" campaign: "straight up? no bull" *Public Health Rep* **114**(6): 522-7.

Arnett, J. (2001). Conceptions of the transition to adulthood: perspectives from adolescence through midlife. *Journal of Adult Development* **8**:133-143.

Arrendondo, E., et al. (2006). Association of a traditional vs. shared meal decision-making and preparation style with eating behavior of Hispanic women in San Diego County. *J Am Diet Assoc* **106**:38-45.

Asfaw, A. (2006). "The Role of Food Price Policy in Determining the Prevalence of Obesity: Evidence from Egypt." *Review of Agricultural Economics* **28**(3): 305-312.

Atkinson, E. (1896). *The science of nutrition; treatise upon the science of nutrition. The Aladdin oven, invented by Edward Atkinson; what it is, what it does, how it does it. Dietaries carefully computed under the direction of Ellen H. Richards. Tests of the slow methods of cooking in the Aladdin oven, by Mary H. Abel and Maria Daniell, with instructions and recipes. Nutritive values of food materials, collated from the writings of W. O. Atwater. Appendix: letters and reports.*

Ayala, G. et al. (2008). "A systematic review of the relationship between acculturation and diet among Latinos in the United States: implications for future research." *J Am Diet Assoc* **108**(8): 1330-44.

Baik, I. et al. (2000). "Adiposity and mortality in men." *Am J Epidemiol* **152**(3): 264-71.

Bandura, A. (1977). *Social Learning Theory*. Englewood Cliffs, NJ, Prentice-Hall.

Bandura, A. (2004). "Health promotion by social cognitive means." *Health Education and Behavior* **31**:143-164.

Baranowski, T. et al. (2003). "Are current health behavioral change models helpful in guiding prevention of weight gain efforts?" *Obesity Research* **11**: 23S-43S.

Baranowski, T. et al. (1999). "Psychosocial Correlates of Dietary Intake: Advancing Dietary Intervention." *Annual Review of Nutrition* **19**: 17-40.

Barnes, A. et al. (2007). Weight loss maintenance in African-American women: Focus group results and questionnaire development. *Soc Gen Intern Med* **22**:915-922.

Bauer, K et al. (2004). "How can we stay healthy when you're throwing all of this in front of us?" Findings from focus groups and interviews in middle schools on environmental influences on nutrition and physical activity. *Health Educ Behav* **31**:34-46.

Baum, C. and Ford, W. (2004). "The wage effects of obesity: a longitudinal study." *Health Econ* **13**(9): 885-99.

Beaulac, J. et al. (2009). "A systematic review of food deserts, 1966-2007." *Prev Chronic Dis* **6**(3): A105.

Bech-Larsen, T. and Grunert, K. (2003). "The perceived healthiness of functional foods. A conjoint study of Danish, Finnish and American consumers' perception of functional foods." *Appetite* **40**(1): 9-14.

Becker, H. (1974). "The Health Belief Model and personal health behavior." *Health Education Monographs* **2**: 324-473.

Becker, K. and Rasmussen, H. (2002). "The New Thrifty Food Plan." *Nutr Clin Care* **5**(4): 199-202.

Bekker, M. et al. (2004). "Effects of negative mood induction and impulsivity on self-perceived emotional eating." *Int J Eat Disord* **36**(4): 461-9.

Bellisle, F. et al. (1988). "Obesity and food intake in children: evidence for a role of metabolic and/or behavioral daily rhythms." *Appetite* **11**(2): 111-8.

Bennett, G. et al. (2007). Immigration and obesity among lower income blacks. *Obesity* **15**:1391-1394.

Benton, D. (2004). Role of parents in the determination of food preferences of children and the development of obesity. *International Journal of Obesity* **28**: 858-869.

Berenson, G. (1986). *Causation of Cardiovascular Risk Factors in Children: Perspectives on Cardiovascular Risk in Early Life*. New York, Raven Press.

Berenson, G. et al. (1980). *Cardiovascular Risk Factors in Children: The Early Natural History of Atherosclerosis and Essential Hypertension*. New York, Oxford University Press.

Berman, W. and Sperling, M. (1991). "Parental attachment and emotional distress in the transition to college." *Journal of Youth and Adolescence* **20**: 427-440.

Birch, L. and Davison, K. (2001). "Family environmental factors influencing the developing behavioral controls of food intake and childhood overweight." *Pediatric Clinics of North America* **48**: 893-907.

Blixen, C. et al. (2006). Values and beliefs about obesity and weight reduction among African American and Causcasian women. *J Trascult Nurs* **17**:290-297.

Block, J. et al. (2004). Fast food, race/ethnicity, and income: a geographic analysis. *Am J Prev Med* **27**(3):211-7.

Bocquier, A. et al. (2005). "Overweight and obesity: knowledge, attitudes, and practices of general practitioners in france." *Obes Res* **13**(4): 787-95.

Boddiger, D. (2007). "Boosting biofuel crops could threaten food security." *Lancet* **370**(9591): 923-4.

Bodor, J. et al. (2008). Neighborhood fruit and vegetable availability and consumption: the role of small food stores in an urban environment. *Public Health Nutr* **11**:413-420.

Booth, K. et al. (2005). "Obesity and the built environment." *J Am Diet Assoc* **105**(5 Suppl 1): S110-7.

Booth-Butterfield, S. and Reger, B. (2004).The message changes belief and the rest is theory: the "1% or less" milk campaign and reasoned action. *Prev Med* **39**(3):581-8.

Bowman, S. et al. (2004). "Effects of fast-food consumption on energy intake and diet quality among children in a National Household Survey." *Pediatrics* **113**(1): 112-118.

Boyd-Orr, J. et al. (1937). *Food, health and income: report on a survey of adequacy of diet in relation to income.* London, Macmillan.

Boynton-Jarrett, R. et al. (2003). Impact of television viewing patterns on fruit and vegetable consumption among adolescents. *Pediatrics* **112**(6 Pt 1):1321-6.

Braus, P. (1995). Selling good behavior. *Am Demogr* **17**(11):60-4.

Brecher, S. et al. (2000). "Status of nutrition labeling, health claims, and nutrient content claims for processed foods: 1997 Food Label and Package Survey." *J Am Diet Assoc* **100**(9): 1057-62.

Brett, J. et al. (2002). Using ethnography to improve intervention design. *Am J Health Promot* **16**:331-40.

Bronner, Y. et al. (1999). "Early introduction of solid foods among urban African-American participatns in WIC." *Journal of the American Dietetic Association* **99**: 457-461.

Brookes, R. (2000). "Creating effective social marketing: let your customer be your guide." *Educ Update* **4**(4): 1-3.

Brown, D. and Tammineni, S. (2009). Managing sales of beverages in schools to preserve profits and improve children's nutrition intake in 15 Mississippi schools. *J Am Diet Assoc* **109**:2036-2042.

Brown, C. et al. (2000). "Body mass index and the prevalence of hypertension and dyslipidemia." *Obes Res* **8**(9): 605-19.

Brug, J. (2006). "Order is needed to promote linear or quantum changes in nutrition and physical activity behaviors: A reaction to 'A chaotic view of behavior change' by Resnicow and Vaughan." *International Journal of Behavioral Nutrition and Physical Activity* **3**: 29-32.

Brummett, B. et al. (2008). "Personality as a predictor of dietary quality in spouses during midlife." *Behavioral Medicine* **34**(1): 5-10.

Bryant, E. et al. (2008). "Disinhibition: its effects on appetite and weight regulation." *Obes Rev* **9**(5): 409-19.

Bungum, T. et al. (2003). "The relationship of body mass index, medical costs, and job absenteeism." *Am J Health Behav* **27**(4): 456-62.

Burke, N. et al. (2009). "The path to active living: physical activity through community design in Somerville, Massachusetts." *Am J Preve Med* **37**(6 Suppl 2): S386-94.

Burke, V. et al. (2005). "Predictors of body mass index and associations with cardiovascular risk factors in Australian children: a prospective cohort study." *Int J Obes (Lond)* **29**(1): 15-23.

Burton, W. et al. (1999). "The costs of body mass index levels in an employed population." *Stat Bull Metrop Insur Co* **80**(3): 8-14.

Byrd-Bredbenner, C. and Finckenor, M. (2000). "Putting The Transtheoretical Model Into Practice With Type 2 Diabetes Mellitus Patients." *Topics in Clinical Nutrition* **15**: 44-58.

Caballero, B. and Popkin, B. (2002). Introduction. In: The Nutrition Transition: Diet and Disease in the Developing World, *Academic Press*, London, UK, pp. 1–5.

Cade, J. et al. (1999). "Costs of a healthy diet: analysis from the UK Women's Cohort Study." *Public Health Nutr* **2**(4): 505-12.

Caillavet, F. et al. (2006). L'alimentation des populations défavorisées en France: synthèse des travaux dans les domaines économique, sociologique et nutritionnel. *Les travaux 2005-2006 de l'Observatoire National de la Pauvreté et de l'Exclusion Sociale.* Paris, Observatoire National de la Pauvreté et de l'Exclusion Sociale.

Calle, E. et al. (2003). "Overweight, obesity, and mortality from cancer in a prospectively studied cohort of U.S. adults." *N Engl J Med* **348**(17): 1625-38.

Campbell, K. et al. (2006) Family food environment and dietary behaviors likely to promote fatness in 5-6 year-old children. *International Journal of Obesity*

Cancer Prevention Research Center and University of Rhode Island. (undated). "Detailed Overview of the Transtheoretical Model." from http://www.uri.edu/research/cprc/ TTM/detailedoverview.htm.

Caraher, M. et al. (1998). "PAPERS - Access to healthy foods: Part I. Barriers to accessing healthy foods: Differentials by gender, social class, income and mode of transport." *The Health Education Journal* **57**(3): 191.

Casey, A. et al. (2008). "Impact of the food environment and physical activity environment on behaviors and weight status in rural U.S. communities." *Prev Med* **47**(6): 600-4.

Cassady, D. et al. (2007). "Is price a barrier to eating more fruits and vegetables for low-income families?" *J Am Diet Assoc* **107**(11): 1909-15.

Centers for Disease Control and Prevention (2006). Research to practice series No. 2: portion size. Atlanta, GA.

Center for Nutrition Policy and Promotion (U.S.) (2005). MyPyramid steps to a healthier you. [Washington, D.C.], U.S. Dept. of Agriculture, Center for Nutrition Policy and Promotion.

Center for Science in the Public Interest, "Food marketing to children." Retrieved February 27, 2010, from http://www.cspinet.org/new/pdf/food_marketing_to_children.pdf.

Center for Disease Prevention (2008). "Prevalence of overweight, obesity and extreme obesity among adults: United States, trends 1960-62 through 2005-2006." Retrieved January 22, 2010, from http://www.cdc.gov/nchs/data/hestat/overweight/overweight_adult.htm.

Center for Disease Prevention, (2009). "Differences in prevalence of obesity among black, white, and Hispanic adults - United States, 2006-2008." *MMWR* **58**(27).

Center for Disease Prevention (2009). "Overweight and obesity: causes and consequences."Retrieved February 17, 2010, from http://www.cdc.gov/obesity/causes/index.html.

Cerin, E. et al. (2009). "Testing theories of dietary behavior change in youth using the mediating variable model with intervention programs." *Journal of Nutrition Education and Behavior* **41**: 309-318.

Cerin, E. and Leslie, E. (2008). "How socio-economic status contributes to participation in leisure-time physical activity." *Soc Sci Med* **66**(12): 2596-609.

Chang, M. et al. (2005). Predictors of fat intake behavior differ between normal-weight and obese WIC mothers. *Am J Health Promot* **19**:269-277.

Chang, M. et al. (2008). Motivators and barriers to healthful eating and physical activity among low-income overweight and obese mothers. *J Am Diet Assoc* **108**:1023-1028.

Chang, M. et al. (2008). Self-efficacy and dietary fat reduction behaviors in obese African-American and white mothers. *Obesity* **16**: 992-1001.

Chatterjee, N. et al. (2005). Perspectives on obesity and barriers to control from workers at a community center serving low-income Hispanic children and families. *J Comm Health Nurs* **22**:23-36.

Cheadle, A. et al. (1993). "Can measures of the grocery store environment be used to track community-level dietary changes?" *Prev Med* **22**(3): 361-72.

Christou, D. et al. (2005). "Fatness is a better predictor of cardiovascular disease risk factor profile than aerobic fitness in healthy men." *Circulation* **111**(15): 1904-14.

Clemens, L. et al. (1999). "The effect of eating out on quality of diet in premenopausal women." *J Am Diet Assoc* **99**(4): 442-4.

Colby, S. et al. (2009). What changes when we move? A transnational exploration of dietary acculturation. *Eco of Food and Nutr* **48**:327-343.

Committee on Public (2001). "Children, adolescents, and television." *Pediatrics* **107**(2): 423-426.

Connors, M. et al. (2001). Managing values in personal food systems. *Appetite* **36**(3):189-200.

Consumer Expenditure Survey Anthology (2008). Washington DC.

Coon, K. et al. (2001). Relationships between use of television during meals and children's food consumption patterns. *Pediatrics* **107** (1).

Coon, K. et al. (2001). "Relationships between use of television during meals and children's food consumption patterns." *Pediatrics* **107**(1): E7.

Courneya, K. and Hellsten, L. (1998). "Personality correlates of exercise behavior,motives, barriers, and preferences: An application of the five-factor model." *Personality and Individual Differences* **24**: 625-633.

Cowburn, G. and Stockley, L. (2005). "Consumer understanding and use of nutrition labeling: a systematic review." *Public Health Nutr* **8**(1): 21-8.

Cox, B. et al. (1997). "Association of anthropometric indices with elevated blood pressure in British adults." *Int J Obes Relat Metab Disord* **21**(8): 674-80.

Crespo, C. et al. (2000). Race/ethnicity, social class and their relation to physical inactivity during leisure time: results from the Third National Health and Nutrition Examination Survey, 1988–1994. *Am J Prev Med*. 2000; 18 (1): 46-53.

Crespo, C. et al. (2001). "Acculturation and leisure-time physical inactivity in Mexican-American adults: results from NHANES III, 1988-1994." *Am J Public Health* **91**(8): 1254-1257.

Crespo C. J., Smit E., Carter-Pokras O., Andersen R. Acculturation andleisure-time physical inactivity in Mexican American adujlts: results from NHANES III, 1988-1994. *Am J Public Health*. 2001;91:1254-1257.

Croll, J. et al. (2001). Healthy eating: what does it mean to adolescents? *J Nutr Educ* **33**:193-198.

Cummins, S. (2003). "The local food environment and health: some reflections from the United kingdom." *Am J Public Health* **93**(4): 521; author reply 521-2.

Dallongeville, J. et al. (2001). "Association between nutrition knowledge and nutritional intake in middle-aged men from Northern France." *Public Health Nutr* **4**(1): 27-33.

Dammann, K. and Smith, C. (2009). Factors affecting low-income women's food choices and the perceived impact of dietary intake and socioeconomic status on their health and weight. *J Nutr Educ Behav* **41**:242-253.

Darmon, N. et al. (2004). "Energy-dense diets are associated with lower diet costs: a community study of French adults." *Public Health Nutrition* **7**(1): 21-27.

Darmon, N. and Drewnowski, A. (2008). "Does social class predict diet quality?" *American Journal of Clinical Nutrition* **87**(5): 1107-1117.

Darmon, N. et al. (2002). "A cost constraint alone has adverse effects on food selection and nutrient density: an analysis of human diets by linear programming." *J Nutr* **132**(12): 3764-71.

Darmon, N. et al. (2006). "Impact of a cost constraint on nutritionally adequate food choices for French women: an analysis by linear programming." *J Nutr Educ Behav* **38**(2): 82-90.

Dave, J. et al. (2009). Associations among food insecurity acculturation, demographic factors, and fruit and vegetable intake at home in Hispanic children. *J Am Diet Assoc* **109**:697-701.

Davis, B. and Carpenter, C. (2009). "Proximity of fast-food restaurants to schools and adolescent obesity." *Am J Public Health* **99**(3): 505-510.

Davis, G. and You, W. (2010). The Thrifty Food Plan is not thrifty when labor cost is considered. *J Nutr* **140**(4):854-7.

de Bruijn, G. et al. (2005). "Is personality related to fruit and vegetable intake and physical activity in adolescents?" *Health Education Research* **20**(6): 635-644.

de Pee, S. et al. (1998). Impact of a social marketing campaign promoting dark-green leafy vegetables and eggs in central Java, Indonesia. *Int J Vitam Nutr Res* **68**(6):389-98.

deVries, H. et al. (2005). "The general public's information needs and perceptions regarding hereditary cancer: an application of the Integrated Change Model." *Patient Education and Counseling* **56**: 154-165.

Dharod, J. (2004). Influence of the Fight BAC! food safety campaign on an urban Latino population in Connecticut. *J Nutr Educ Behav* **36**(3):128-32.

Dietary guidelines for Americans (2005). 6th edition. US Department of Health and Human Services and US Department of Agriculture. http://www.health.gov/dietaryguidelines/dga2005/document/pdf/DGA2005.pdf. Accessed March 9, 2010.

Dixon, H. et al. (1998) Public reaction to Victoria's "2 Fruit 'n' 5 Veg Every Day" campaign and reported consumption of fruit and vegetables. *Prev Med* **27**(4):572-82.

Dowler, E. and Dobson, B. (1997). "Nutrition and poverty in Europe: an overview." *Proc Nutr Soc* **56**(1A): 51-62.

Dreon, D. et al. (1988). "Dietary fat:carbohydrate ratio and obesity in middle-aged men." *Am J Clin Nutr* **47**(6): 995-1000.

Drewnowski, A. and Darmon, N. (2005). "Food choices and diet costs: an economic analysis." *Journal of Nutrition* **135**(4): 900-904.

Drewnowski, A. and Darmon, N. (2005). "The economics of obesity: dietary energy density and energy cost." *Am J Clin Nutr* **82**(1 Suppl): 265S-273S.

Drewnowski, A. et al. (2004). "Replacing fats and sweets with vegetables and fruits—a question of cost." *Am J Public Health* **94**(9): 1555-9.

Duffey, K. et al. (2008). Birthplace is associated with more adverse dietary profiles for US-born than for foreign-born Latino adults. *J Nutr* **138**:2428-2435.

Dunstan, D. et al. (2002). "High-intensity resistance training improves glycemic control in older patients with type 2 diabetes." *Diabetes Care* **25**(10): 1729-36.

Edelstein, S. et al. (1992). "Increased meal frequency associated with decreased cholesterol concentrations; Rancho Bernardo, CA, 1984-1987." *Am J Clin Nutr* **55**(3): 664-9.

Edwards, P. and Roberts, I. (2008). "Transport policy is food policy." *Lancet* **371**(9625): 1661.

Eikenberry, N and Smith, C. (2004). Healthful eating: Perceptions, motivations, barriers, and promoters in low-income Minnesota communities. *J Am Diet Assoc* **104**:1158-1161.

Evans, N. et al. (1995). Adolescents' perceptions of their peers' health norms. *Am J Public Health* **85**:1064-9.

Eyler, A. et al. (1998). Physical activity and minority women: a qualitative study. *Health Educ Behav* **25**: 640-652.

Evans, A. et al. (2009). "Parental feeding practices and concerns related to child underweight, picky eating, and using food to calm differ according to ethnicity/race, acculturation, and income." Matern Child Health J Published online: 22 Sept 2009.

Eyler, A. et al. (1999). Physical activity social support and middle-and older-aged minority women: results from a US survey. *Soc Sci Med* **49**:781-789.

Eyler, A. and Vest, J. (2002). Environmental and policy factors related to physical activity in rural white women. *Women Health* **36**: 111-121.

Fabricatore, A. and Wadden, T. (2004). "Psychological aspects of obesity." *Clin Dermatol* **22**(4): 332-7.

Fabry, P. (1970). "Significance of meal frequency in man." *N Y State J Med* **70**(5): 668-70.

Fabry, P. and Tepperman, J. (1970). "Meal frequency—a possible factor in human pathology." *Am J Clin Nutr* **23**(8): 1059-68.

Fabry, P. et al. (1966). "Effect of meal frequency in schoolchildren. Changes in weight-height proportion and skinfold thickness." *Am J Clin Nutr* **18**(5): 358-61.

FAO (2006). *The double burden of malnutrition: case studies from six developing countries.* FAO food and nutrition paper, 84, 2006. Rome: Food and Agriculture Organization of the United Nations.

FAO (2009). "1.02 billion people hungry (press release)." Retrieved November 2009, from http://www.fao.org/news/story/en/item/20568/icode/. Farm subsidy data, 2006. (2008) Washington, Environmental Working Group: News Release.

Ferrara, C. et al. (2004). "Metabolic effects of the addition of resistive to aerobic exercise in older men." *Int J Sport Nutr Exerc Metab* **14**(1): 73-80.

Ferrie, J. et al. (1998). "An Uncertain Future: The Health Effects of Threats to Employment Security in White-Collar Men and Women." *American Journal of Public Health* **88**(7): 1030-1036.

Field, A., E. Coakley, et al. (2001). "Impact of overweight on the risk of developing common chronic diseases during a 10-year period." *Archives of Internal Medicine,* **161**(13), 1581-6.

Fields, D. et al. (2002). "Body-composition assessment via air-displacement plethysmography in adults and children: a review." *Am J Clin Nutr* **75**(3): 453-67.

Finkelstein, E. et al. (2005). "Economic causes and consequences of obesity." *Annu Rev Public Health* **26**: 239-57.

Finkelstein, E. et al. (2004). "State-level estimates of annual medical expenditures attributable to obesity." *Obes Res* **12**(1): 18-24.

Fisher, J. and Neumark-Sztainer, D. (2003). "Factors influencing eating behaviors." *Dairy Council Digest* **74**(3): 13-18.

Fiske, A. and Cullen, K. (2004). "Effects of promotional materials on vending sales of low-fat items in teachers' lounges." *J Am Diet Assoc* **104**(1): 90-3.

Fitzgerald, N. and Spaccarotella, K. (2009). Barriers to a healthy lifestyle: from individuals to public policy- an ecological perspective. *Journal of Extension* **47**(1).

Fitzgerald, N. et al. (2006). "Acculturation, socioeconomic status, obesity and lifestyle factors among low-income Puerto Rican women in Connecticut, U.S., 1998-1999." *Rev Panam Salud Publica* **19**(5): 306-13.

Fitzgibbon, M and Stolley, M. (2004). Environmental changes may be needed for prevention of overweight in minority children. *Pediatr Ann* **33**:45-9.

Flegal, K. et al. (2004). "Methods of calculating deaths attributable to obesity." *Am J Epidemiol* **160**(4): 331-8.

Flegal, K. et al. (2005). "Excess deaths associated with underweight, overweight, and obesity." *Jama* **293**(15): 1861-7.

Flegal, K. et al. (2006). "Weight and mortality." *Hypertension* 47(2): e6; author reply e6-7.

Flegal, K. et al. (2004). "Fraction of premature deaths in the Canadian population that were attributable to overweight and obesity." *Can J Public Health* **95**(3): 235; author reply 235.

Flegal, K. et al. (2010). "Prevalence and trends in obesity among US adults, 1999-2008." *JAMA* **303**(3): 235-241.

Foerster, S. et al. (1995). California's "5 a day—for better health!" campaign: an innovative population-based effort to effect large-scale dietary change. *Am J Prev Med* **11**(2):124-31.

Fogelholm, M. (2009). "Physical activity, fitness and fatness: relations to mortality, morbidity and disease risk factors. A systematic review." *Obes Rev.*

Fontaine, K. et al. (2003). "Years of life lost due to obesity." *Jama* **289**(2): 187-93.

Food Marketing Institute. (2006). *U.S. Grocery Shopping Trends 2006*. Washington, DC: Food Marketing Institute.

Food security in the United States: An assessment of the measure. US Department of Agriculture Economic Research Service. Available at: http://www.ers.usda.gov/Briefing/FoodSecurity/nassummary.htm. Accessed March 9, 2010.

Ford, E. et al. (2001). "Self-reported body mass index and health related quality of life: findings from the Behavioral Risk Factor Surveillance System." *Obes Res* **9**(1): 21-31.

Foster, G. et al. (2003). "Primary care physicians' attitudes about obesity and its treatment." *Obes Res* **11**(10): 1168-77.

Franco, M. et al. (2009) Availability of healthy foods and dietary patterns: the Multi-Ethnic Study of Atherosclerosis. **89**:897-904.

Fredrickson, B. (2000). "Cultivating Positive Emotions to Optimize Health and Well-Being." *Prevention & Treatment* **3**: Article 0001a.

Freedman, D. et al. (2007). "Childhood overweight and family income." *Med Gen Med* **9**(2): 26.

Freimuth, V. et al. (1988). "Health advertising: prevention for profit." *Am J Public Health* **78**(5): 557-61.

French, S. (2003). "Pricing effects on food choices." *J Nutr* **133**(3): 841S-843S.

French, S. et al. (2001). "Pricing and promotion effects on low-fat vending snack purchases: the CHIPS Study." *Am J Public Health* **91**(1): 112-7.

Fullmer, S. et al. (1991). "Consumers' knowledge, understanding, and attitudes toward health claims on food labels." *J Am Diet Assoc* **91**(2): 166-71.

Galasso, P. et al. (2005). Barriers to medical nutrition therapy in black women with diabetes mellitus. *The Diabetes Educator* **31**: 719.

Galobardes, B. et al. (2007). "Measuring socioeconomic position in health research." *Br Med Bull* **81-82**: 21-37.

Gelber, R. et al. (2005). "Association between body mass index and CKD in apparently healthy men." *Am J Kidney Dis* **46**(5): 871-80.

Geliebter, A.. and Aversa, A. (2003). "Emotional eating in overweight, normal weight, and underweight individuals." *Eat Behav* **3**(4): 341-7.

Geronimus, A. (2001). "Understanding and Eliminating Racial Inequalities in Women's Health in the United States: The Role of the Weathering Conceptual Framework." *Journal of the American Medical Women's Association* **56**: 133-136.

Gielen, A. et al. Eds. (2008). *Using the PRECEDE-PROCEED Model to Apply Health Behavior Theories*. Health Behavior and Health Education. Theory, Research, and Practice. San Francisco, Jossey-Bass.

Gilbert, L. (2000). "The functional food trend: what's next and what Americans think about eggs." *J Am Coll Nutr* **19**(5 Suppl): 507S-512S.

Giles-Corti, B. and Donovan, J. (2002). "Socioeconomic status differences in recreational physical activity levels and real and perceived access to a supportive physical environment." *Prev Med* **35**(6): 601-11.

Giles-Corti, B. et al. (2003). "Environmental and lifestyle factors associated with overweight and obesity in Perth, Australia." *Am J Health Promot* **18**(1): 93-102.

Giskes, K. et al. (2007). "A systematic review of associations between environmental factors, energy and fat intakes among adults: is there evidence for environments that encourage obesogenic dietary intakes?" *Public Health Nutr* **10**(10): 1005-17.

Glanz, K. et al. (1998). Why Americans eat what they do: taste, nutrition, cost, convenience, an weight control concerns as influences on food consumption. *J Am Diet Assoc* **98**:1118-1126.

Glanz, K. et al. (2005). Healthy Nutrition Environments Concepts and Measures. 2005. *Am J Health Promot* **19**(5):330-333.

Glanz, K. et al., Eds. (2008). *Theory, research, and practice in health behavior and health education.* Health Behavior and Health Educ. Theory, Research, and Practice. San Francisco, Jossey-Bass.

Glanz, K. et al. (2002). Health Behavior and Health Education. Theory, Research and Practice. San Francisco: Wiley & Sons.

Godfrey, J. (2008).Toward optimal health: Dr. Kelly Brownell discusses the influence of the environment on obesity. *Journal of Women's Health* **17** (3):325-330.

Goel, M. et al. (2004). "Obesity among US immigrant subgroups by duration of residence." *JAMA* **292**: 2860-67.

Gollwitzer, P. (1996). Volitional Benefits of Planning. *The psychology of action.* P. Gollwitzer and J. Bargh. New York, Guilford Press: 287-312.

Goodman, E. and Whitaker, R. (2002). "A prospective study of the role of depression in the development and persistence of adolescent obesity." *Pediatrics* **110**(3): 497-504.

Gordon-Larsen, P. et al. (2004). Longitudinal physical activity and sedentary behavior trends: adolescence to adulthood. *Am J Prev Med* **27**:277-83.

Gordon-Larsen, P. (2009). "Entry into romantic partnership is associated with obesity." *Obesity* **17**(7): 1441-1447.

Goulet, J. et al. (2008). "A Nutritional Intervention Promoting a Mediterranean Food Pattern Does Not Affect Total Daily Dietary Cost in North American Women in Free-Living Conditions." *J. Nutr.* **138**(1): 54-59.

Gray, V. et al. (2005). "Dietary acculturation of Hispanic immigrants in Mississippi." *Salud Publica Mex* **47**(5): 351-60.

Greaney, M. et al. (2009) College Students' Barriers and Enablers for Healthful Weight Management: A Qualitative Study. *J Nutr Educ Behav* **41**:281-286.

Green, L. and Kreuter, M. (2005). *Health promotion planning: An educational and ecological approach.* New York, McGraw-Hill.

Greenberg, M. and Renne, J. (2005). Where does walkability matter the most? An environmental justice interpretation of New Jersey data. *Journal of Urban Health* **82**:90-100.

Gregson, J. et al. (2001). System, environmental, and policy changes: using the social-ecological model as a framework for evaluating nutrition education and social marketing programs with low-income audiences. *J Nutr Educ* **33** Suppl 1:S4-15.

Guenther, P. et al. (2006). "Healthy Eating Index-2005." Retrieved February 20, 2010, from http://www.cnpp.usda.gov/Publications/HEI/healthyeatingindex2005factsheet.pdf.

Guenther, P. et al. (2008). "Diet quality of Americans in 1994-96 and 2001-02 as measured by the Healthy Eating Index 2005." Retrieved February 20, 2010, from http://www.cnpp.usda.gov/Publications/NutritionInsights/Insight37.pdf.

Guo, S. et al. (1994). "The predictive value of childhood body mass index values for overweight at age 35 y." *American Journal of Clinical Nutrition* **59**(4): 810-819.

Guthrie, J. and Lin, B. (2002). Overview of the diets of lower-and higher-income elderly and their food assistance options. *Journal of Nutrition Education and Behavior* **34**(supp1):S31-S41.

Haapalahti, M. et al. (2003). "Meal patterns and food use in 10-to 11- year-old Finnish children." *Public Health Nutrition* **6**(4): 365-370.

Haines, J. et al. (2006). "Weight-teasing and disordered eating behaviors in adolescents: Longitudinal findings from Project EAT (Eating Among Teens)." *Pediatrics* **117**: e209-215.

Halford, J. et al. (2004). Effect of television advertisements for foods on food consumption in children. *Appetite* **42**(2):221-5.

Hampl, S. et al. (2007). "Resource utilization and expenditures for overweight and obese children." *Arch Pediatr Adolesc Med* **161**(1): 11-4.

Harnack, L. et al. (1999). Diet and physical activity patterns of Lakota Indian adults. *J Am Diet Assoc* **99**:829-835.

Harnack, L. et al. (1999). Diet and physical activity patterns of urban American Indian women. **13** (4): 233-236.

Harris, J. et al. (2010). "Marketing foods to children and adolescents: licensed characters and other promotions on packaged foods in the supermarket." *Public Health Nutr* **13**(3): 409-17.

Harrison, K. and Marske, A. (2005). "Nutritional content of foods advertised during the television programs children watch most." *Am J Public Health* **95**(9): 1568-74.

Hart, K. et al. (2003). Promoting healthy diet and exercise patterns amongst primary school children: a qualitative investigation of parental perspectives. *J Hum Nutr Diet* **16**:89-96.

Harvey, E. and Hill, A. (2001). "Health professionals' views of overweight people and smokers." *Int J Obes Relat Metab Disord* **25**(8): 1253-61.

Hays, N. et al. (2002). "Eating behavior correlates of adult weight gain and obesity in healthy women aged 55-65 y." *Am J Clin Nutr* **75**(3): 476-83.

He, M. et al. (2001). "Body fat determination by dual energy X-ray absorptiometry and its relation to body mass index and waist circumference in Hong Kong Chinese." *Int J Obes Relat Metab Disord* **25**(5): 748-52.

Heitmann, B. et al. (2000). "Mortality associated with body fat, fat-free mass and body mass index among 60-year-old swedish men-a 22-year follow-up. The study of men born in 1913." *Int J Obes Relat Metab Disord* **24**(1): 33-7.

Hendler, R. et al. (1995). "The effects of weight reduction to ideal body weight on body fat distribution." *Metabolism* **44**(11): 1413-6.

Hendrix, S. et al. (2008). Fruit and vegetable intake and knowledge increased following a community-based intervention in older adults in Georgia senior centers. *J Nutr for the Elderly* **27**:155-178.

Hetherington, E. (1999). *Child Psychology*. Boston, MA, McGraw-Hill College Inc.

Hildebrand, D. and Betts, N. (2009). Assessment of Stage of Change, decisional balance, self efficacy, and use of processes of change of low-income parents for increasing servings of fruits and vegetables to preschool-aged children. *J Nutr Educ Behav* **41**:110-119.

Henderson, V. and Kelly, B. (2005). Food advertising in the age of obesity: content analysis of food advertising on general market and African American television. *J Nutr Educ Behav* **37**(4):191-6.

Hill, J. and Peters, J. (1998). "Environmental contributions to the obesity epidemic." *Science* **280**(5368): 1371-4.

Himmelgreen, D. et al. (2004). "The longer you stay, the bigger you get: length of time and language use in the U.S. are associated with obesity in Puerto Rican women." *Am J Phys Anthropol* **125**(1): 90-6.

Himmelgreen, D. et al. (2007). "I don't make the soups anymore: pre- to post-migration dietary and lifestyle changes among Latinos living in west-Central Florida." *Ecol Food Nutr* **46**: 427-444.

Hjartaker, A. et al. (2005). "Body mass index and mortality in a prospectively studied cohort of Scandinavian women: the women's lifestyle and health cohort study." *Eur J Epidemiol* **20**(9): 747-54.

Horacek, T. and Betts, N. (1998). "Students cluster into 4 groups according to the factors influencing their dietary intake." *Journal of the American Dietetic Association* **98**: 14641467.

Horowitz, C. et al. (2004). Barriers to buying healthy foods for people with diabetes: evidence of environmental disparities. *Am J Public Health* **94**: 1549-1554.

Hou, L. et al. (2006). "Body mass index and colon cancer risk in Chinese people: menopause as an effect modifier." *Eur J Cancer* **42**(1): 84-90.

Hsu, C. et al. (2006). "Body mass index and risk for end-stage renal disease." *Ann Intern Med* **144**(1): 21-8.

Huhman, M. et al. (2005). Effects of a mass media campaign to increase physical activity among children: year-1 results of the VERB campaign. *Pediatrics* **116**(2):e277-84.

Humphries, J. (2009). "The cost of obesity in the United States." Retrieved January 24, 2010, from http://www.executivehm.com/news/cost-of-obesity-in-the-united-states/.

Hunt, L. et al. (2004). "Should "acculturation" be a variable in health research? A critical review of research on US Hispanics." *Soc Sci Med* **59**(5): 973-86.

Ibanez, J. et al. (2005). "Twice-weekly progressive resistance training decreases abdominal fat and improves insulin sensitivity in older men with type 2 diabetes." *Diabetes Care* **28**(3): 662-7.

Inglis, V. (2009). "Does modifying the household food budget predict changes in the healthfulness of purchasing choices among low- and high income women?" *Appetite* **52**(2): 273-9.

Institute of Medicine (2006). Food marketing to children: threat or opportunity? Washington, DC, National Academies Press.

Jabs, J. and Devine, C. (2006). "Time scarcity and food choices: an overview." *Appetite* **47**(2): 196-204.

Jackson, A. and Pollock, M. (1978). "Generalized equations for predicting body density of men." *Br J Nutr* **40**(3): 497-504.

Jackson, A. et al. (1980). "Generalized equations for predicting body density of women." *Med Sci Sports Exerc* **12**(3): 175-81.

Jacobson, M. and Brownell, K. (2000). "Small taxes on soft drinks and snack foods to promote health." *Am J Public Health* **90**(6): 854-7.

James, D. (2004). Factors influencing food choices, dietary intake, and nutrition-related attitudes among African Americans: application of a culturally sensitive model. *Ethn Health* **9**:349-367.

Janssen, I. and Mark, A. (2006). "Separate and combined influence of body mass index and waist circumference on arthritis and knee osteoarthritis." *Int J Obes (Lond)*.

Janssen, I. et al. (2002). "Body mass index, waist circumference, and health risk: evidence in support of current National Institutes of Health guidelines." *Arch Intern Med* **162**(18): 2074-9.

Jeffery, R. et al. (1991). "Socioeconomic status differences in health behaviors related to obesity: the Healthy Worker Project." *Int J Obes* **15**(10): 689-96.

Jeffreys, M. et al. (2004). "Childhood body mass index and later cancer risk: a 50-year follow-up of the Boyd Orr study." *Int J Cancer* **112**(2): 348-51.

Jeffreys, M. et al. (2003). "Body mass index in early and mid-adulthood, and subsequent mortality: a historical cohort study." *Int J Obes Relat Metab Disord* **27**(11): 1391-7.

Jekanowski, M. (1999). Causes and consequences of fast food sales growth. *Food Rev* 11-6.

Jilcott, S. et al. (2007). Perceptions of the community food environment and related influences on food choice among midlife women residing in rural and urban Areas: a qualitative analysis. *Women and Health* **49**: 2, 164-180.

Johnston, E. et al. (2004). "The relation of body mass index to depressive symptoms." *Can J Public Health* **95**(3): 179-83.

Joshi, A. V., D. Day, et al. (2005). "Relationship between obesity and cardiovascular risk factors: findings from a multi-state screening project in the United States." *Curr Med Res Opin* **21**(11): 1755-61.

Kant, A. and Graubard, B. (2004). Eating out in America, 1987-2000: trends and nutritional correlates. *Preventive Medicine* **38**(2):243-249.

Kant, A. and Graubard, B. (2005). "Energy density of diets reported by American adults: association with food group intake, nutrient intake, and body weight." *Int J Obes (Lond)* **29**(8): 950-6.

Katan, M. and de Roos, N. (2003). "Public health. Toward evidence-based health claims for foods." *Science* **299**(5604): 206-7.

Katz, D. The NuVal™ Nutritional Scoring System. Accessed on 11/4/09 from: http://www.nuval.com/

Katzmarzyk, P. et al. (2002). "Adiposity, adipose tissue distribution and mortality rates in the Canada Fitness Survey follow-up study." *Int J Obes Relat Metab Disord* **26**(8): 1054-9.

Katzmarzyk, P. et al. (2001). "Fitness, fatness, and estimated coronary heart disease risk: the HERITAGE Family Study." *Med Sci Sports Exerc* **33**(4): 585-90.

Kearney, J. et al. (1999). Methods used to conduct the pan-European Union survey on consumer attitudes to physical activity, body weight and health. *Public Health Nutr* **2**:79-86.

Kearney, J. and McElhone, S. (1999). "Perceived barriers in trying to eat healthier— results of a pan-EU consumer attitudinal survey." *Br J Nutr* **81 Suppl 2**: S133-7.

Kennedy, E. et al. (1995). "The Healthy Eating Index: design and applications." *J of the Am Dietetic Assoc* **95**(10): 1103-8.

King, A. et al. (2000). Personal and environmental factors associated with physical inactivity among different racial–ethnic groups of U.S. middle-aged and older-aged women. *Hlth Psych* **19**:354-364.

King, K. et al. (2008). Effect of social support on adolescents' perceptions of and engagement in physical activity. *J Phys Act Health* **5**:374-384.

Kiviniemi, M. and Duangdao, K. (2009).Affective associations mediate the influence of cost-benefit beliefs on fruit and vegetable consumptions. *Appetite* **52**: 771-775.

Knip, M. and Akerblom, H. (2005). "Early nutrition and later diabetes risk." *Advanced Experimental Medical Biology* **569**: 142-150.

Kodama, H. et al. (1999). "Gallstone disease risk in relation to body mass index and waist-to-hip ratio in Japanese men." *Int J Obes Relat Metab Disord* **23**(2): 211-6.

Köhler, B. et al. Eds. (1997). *Poverty and food in welfare societies*. Berlin, Ed. Sigma.

Kotler, P. (1997). *Marketing Management:Analysis, Planning, Implementation and Control*. Upper Saddle River, New Jersey, Simon & Schuster.

Kotz, K. and Story, M. (1994). Food advertisements during children's Saturday morning television programming: are they consistent with dietary recommendations? *J Am Diet Assoc* **94**(11):1296-300.

Krebs-Smith, S. et al. (1987). "The effects of variety in food choices on dietary quality." *J Am Diet Assoc* **87**(7): 897-903.

Kreuter, M. et al. (1997). "Do nutrition label readers eat healthier diets? Behavioral correlates of adults' use of food labels." *Am J Prev Med* **13**(4): 277-83.

Kroeber, A. and Kluckhohn, C. (1952). *Culture: A Critical Review of Concepts and Definitions*. Cambridge, MA, Peabody Museum.

Kunkel, D., C. McKinley, et al. (2009) The impact of industry self-regulation on the nutritional quality of foods advertised on television to children. *Children Now.*

Kurth, T. et al. (2002). "Body mass index and the risk of stroke in men." *Arch Intern Med* **162**(22): 2557-62.

Kurth, T. et al. (2005). "Prospective study of body mass index and risk of stroke in apparently healthy women." *Circulation* **111**(15): 1992-8.

Laaksonen, D. et al. (2005). "Physical activity in the prevention of type 2 diabetes: the Finnish diabetes prevention study." *Diabetes* **54**(1): 158-65.

Lamon-Fava, S. et al. (1996). "Impact of body mass index on coronary heart disease risk factors in men and women. The Framingham Offspring Study." *Arterioscler Thromb Vasc Biol* **16**(12): 1509-15.

Langsetmo, L. et al. (2010). "Dietary patterns in Canadian men and women ages 25 and older: relationship to demographics, body mass index, and bone mineral density." *BMC Musculoskeletal Disorders* **11**(1): 20.

Lank NH, Vickery CE, Cotugna N, Shade DD. Food commercials during television soap operas: what is the nutrition message? *J Community Health*. 1992 Dec;17 (6):377-84.

Lara, M. et al. (2005). "Acculturation and Latino health in the United States: a reivew of the literature and its sociopolitical context." *Annu Rev Public Health* **26**: 367-97.

Laraia, B. et al. (2004). Proximity of supermarkets is positively associated with diet quality index for pregnancy. *Prev Med* **39**:869-875.

Larson, N. et al. (2006). Food preparation and purchasing roles among adolescents: Associations with sociodemographic characteristics and diet quality. *J Am Diet Assoc* **106**:211-218.

Larson, N. et al. (2007). "Trends in adolescent fruit and vegetable consumption, 1999-2004: project EAT." *Am J Prev Med* **32**(2): 147-50.

Larson, R. (1990). "The solitary side of life: An examination of the time people spend alone from childhood to old age." *Developmental Review* **10**: 155-183.

Laska, M. et al. (2009). "Latent class analysis of lifestyle characteristics and health risk behaviors among college youth." *Prev Sci* **10**(4): 376-86.

Latner, J. and Stunkard, A. (2003). "Getting worse: the stigmatization of obese children." *Obes Res* **11**(3): 452-6.

Lawson, O. et al. (1995). "The association of body weight, dietary intake, and energy expenditure with dietary restraint and disinhibition." *Obes Res* **3**(2): 153-61.

Lee, S. et al. (2005). "Exercise without weight loss is an effective strategy for obesity reduction in obese individuals with and without Type 2 diabetes." *J Appl Physiol* **99**(3): 1220-5.

Legault, L. et al. (2004). "2000-2001 food label and package survey: an update on prevalence of nutrition labeling and claims on processed, packaged foods." *J Am Diet Assoc* **104**(6): 952-8.

Levy, L. et al. (2000). "How well do consumers understand percentage daily value on food labels?" *Am J Health Promot* **14**(3): 157-60, ii.

Lewis, L. et al. (2005). REACH Coalition of the African Americans Building a Legacy of Health Project. African Americans' access to healthy food options in South Los Angeles restaurants. *Am J Public Health* **95**(4):668-73.

Liese, A. et al. (2007). Food store types, availability, and cost of foods in a rural environment. *J Am Diet Assoc* **107**:1916-1923.

Liou, D. and Bauer, K. (2007). Exploratory investigation of obesity risk and prevention in Chinese Americans. *J Nutr Educ Behav* **39**:134-141.

Lippke, S. and Plotnikoff, R. (2009). "The protection motivation theory within the stages of the transtheoretical model - Stage-specific interplay of variables and prediction of exercise stage transitions." *British Journal of Human Psychology* **14**: 211-229.

Littman, A. et al. (2005). "Effects of physical activity intensity, frequency, and activity type on 10-y weight change in middle-aged men and women." *Int J Obes (Lond)* **29**(5): 524-33.

Lobstein, T. and Dibb, S. (2005). Evidence of a possible link between obesogenic food advertising and child overweight. *Obes Rev* **6**(3):203-8.

Locher, J. et al. Food choice among homebound older adults: motivations and perceived barriers. *J Nutr Health.* 2009;13: 659-664.

Lopez, C. et al. (2009). "Costs of Mediterranean and western dietary patterns in a Spanish cohort and their relationship with prospective weight change." *J Epidemiol Com Hlth* **63**(11): 920-7.

Locher, J. et al. (2009). Food choice among homebound older adults: motivations and perceived barriers. *J Nutr Health* **13**: 659-664.

Lopez-Quintero, C. et al. (2009). Limited English proficiency is a barrier to receipt of advice about physical activity and diet among Hispanics with chronic diseases in the United States. *J Am Diet Assoc* **109**: 1769-1774.

Lorson, B. et al. (2009). Correlates of fruit and vegetable intakes in US children. *J Am Diet Assoc.* **109**:474-478.

Ma, Y. et al. (2003). Association between eating patterns and obesity in a free-living US adult population. *Am J Epidemiol* **158**:85-92.

Maddux, J. (1993). "Social cognitive models of health and exercise behavior: an introduction and review of conceptual issues." *Journal of Applied Sports Psychology* **5**: 116-140.

Mahadevan, M. and Blair, D. (2009). Changes in foods habits of South Indian Hindu Brahmin immigrants in State College, PA. *Eco of Food and Nutr* **48**:404-432.

Maillot, M. et al. (2010). "Are lowest-cost healthful food plans socially acceptable?" *Public Health Nutrition* **In press**.

Maillot, M. et al. (2008). "Nutrient profiling can help identify foods of good nutritional quality for their price: A validation study with linear programming." *Journal of Nutrition* **138**(6): 1107-1113.

Maillot, M. et al. (2007). "Low energy density and high nutritional quality are each associated with higher diet costs in French adults." *American Journal of Clinical Nutrition* **86**(3): 690-696.

Maillot, M. et al. (2007). "Nutrient profiling of food groups can help consumers to select optimal diets at an affordable cost." *Annals of Nutrition and Metabolism* **51**: 328-328.

Maillot, M. et al. (2007). "Nutrient-dense food groups have high energy costs: an econometric approach to nutrient profiling." *J Nutr* **137**(7): 1815-20.

Masse, L. and Anderson, C. (2003). Ethnic differences among correlates of physical activity in women. *Am J Health Promot.* **17**:357-360.

May, A. et al. (2007). "Child-Feeding Strategies Are Associated with Maternal Concern about Children Becoming Overweight, but not Children's Weight Status." *Journal of the American Dietetic Association* **107**(7): 1167-74.

McAllister, M. et al. (1994). "Financial Costs of Healthful Eating: A Comparison of Three Different Approaches." *Journal of Nutrition Education* **26**(3): 131.

McCreedy, M. and Leslie, J. (2009). "Get Active Orlando: changing the built environment to increase physical activity." *Am J Prev Med* **37**(6 Suppl 2): S395-402.

McCrory, M. et al. (1999). "Dietary variety within food groups: association with energy intake and body fatness in men and women." *Am J Clin Nutr* **69**(3): 440-7.

McCrory, M. et al. (1999). "Overeating in America: association between restaurant food consumption and body fatness in healthy adult men and women ages 19 to 80." *Obes Res* **7**(6): 564-71.

McCrory, M. et al. (2000). "Dietary determinants of energy intake and weight regulation in healthy adults." *J Nutr* **130**(2S Suppl): 276S-279S.

McDivitt, J. et al. (1993). The impact of the Healthcom mass media campaign on timely initiation of breastfeeding in Jordan. *Stud Fam Plann* **24**(5):295-309.

McGinnis, J. et al. Ed. (2006). *Food Marketing to Children and Youth Threat or Opportunity?* Institute of Medicine (U.S.). Committee on Food Marketing and the Diets of Children and Youth, National Academy of Sciences.

McLaren, L. (2007). "Socioeconomic Status and Obesity." *Epidemiol Rev* **29**(1): 29-48.

McLaughlin, C. et al. (2003). "An examination of at-home food preparation activity among low-income, food-insecure women." *Journal of the American Dietetic Association* **103**(11): 1506-1512.

McLaughlin, E. (2004). "The dynamics of fresh fruit and vegetable pricing in the supermarket channel." *Prev Med* **39** Suppl 2: S81-7.

Metzner, H. et al. (1977). "The relationship between frequency of eating and adiposity in adult men and women in the Tecumseh Community Health Study." *Am J Clin Nutr* **30**(5): 712-5.

Michella, S. and Slaugh, B. (2000). "Producing and marketing a specialty egg." *Poult Sci* **79**(7): 975-6.

Michels, K. et al. (2008). A study of the importance of education and cost incentives on individual food choices at the Harvard School of Public Health cafeteria. *J Am Coll Nutr* **27**:6-11.

Miller, J. and Coble, K. (2007). "Cheap food policy: Fact or rhetoric?" *Food policy.* **32**(1): 98-111.

Miller, K. et al. (2000). "Comparisons of body image dimensions by race/ethnicity and gender in a university population." *Int J Eat Disord* **27**(3): 310-6.

Miller, Y. and Dunstan, D. (2004). "The effectiveness of physical activity interventions for the treatment of overweight and obesity and type 2 diabetes." *J Sci Med Sport* **7**(1 Suppl): 52-9.

Monsivais, P. and Drewnowski, A. (2007). The rising cost of low-energy-density foods. *J Am Diet Assoc.* **107**: 2071-2076.

Monsivais, A. (2009). "Lower-energy-density diets are associated with higher monetary costs per kilocalorie and are consumed by women of higher socioeconomic status." *Journal of the American Dietetic Association* **In Press**.

Montano, D. and Kasprzyk, D. (2008). Theory of reasoned action, theory of planned behavior, and the integrated behavioral model. *Health Behavior and Health Education. Theory, Research, and Practice.* Glanz, K. et al. San Francisco, Jossey-Bass.

Moore, L. and Diez Roux, A. (2006). Associations of neighborhood characteristics with the location and type of food stores. *Am J Public Health* **96**(2):325-31. Epub 2005 Dec 27.

Morimoto, L. et al. (2002). "Obesity, body size, and risk of postmenopausal breast cancer: the Women's Health Initiative (United States)." *Cancer Causes Control* **13**(8): 741-51.

Morland, K. et al. (2002). Neighborhood characteristics associated with the location of food stores and food service places. *Am J Prev Med.* **22**(1):23-29.

Must, A. et al. (1999). "The disease burden associated with overweight and obesity." *Jama* **282**(16): 1523-9.

National Institutes of Health, National Heart, Lung, and Blood Institute. (1998, September). "Clinical Guidelines on the Identification, Evaluation, and Treatment of Overweight and Obesity in Adults—The Evidence Report." from http://www.nhlbi.nih.gov/guidelines/obesity/ob_gdlns.htm.

Nelson, M. et al. (2008). "Associations between credit card debt, stress, and leading health risk behaviors among college students." *American Journal of Health Promotion* **22**(6): 400-407.

Nelson, M. et al. (2008). "Emerging adulthood and college-aged youth: An overlooked age for weight-related behavior change." *Obesity* **16**(10): 2205-11.

Neumark-Sztainer, D. et al. (2003). Family meal patterns: Associations with sociodemographic characteristics and improved dietary intake among adolescents. *J Am Diet Assoc* **103**:317-322.

Neumark-Sztainer, D. et al. Correlates of fruit and vegetable intake among adolescents: Findings from Project EAT. *Prev Med.* 2003;**37**:198-208.

Neumark-Sztainer, D. (2003). "Childhood and adolescent obesity: An ecological perspective." *Pediatric Basics* **101**: 13-18, 20.

Neumark-Sztainer, D. et al. (1999). Factors influencing food choices of adolescents: findings from focus-group discussions with adolescents. *J am Diet Assoc* **99**:929-937.

Neumark-Sztainer, D. et al. (2002). "Weight-teasing among adolescents: Correlations with weight status and disordered eating behaviors." *International Journal of Obesity and Related Metabolic Disorders* **26**(1): 123-131.

Nicklas, T. et al. (1998). "Impact of breakfast consumption on nutritional adequacy of the diets of young adults in Bogalusa, Louisiana: ethnic and gender contrasts." *J Am Diet Assoc* **98**(12): 1432-8.

Nielsen, S. and Popkin, B. (2003). Patterns and trends in food portion sizes, 1977-1998. *JAMA* **289**:450-453.

Nielsen, S. and Popkin, B (2004). "Changes in beverage intake between 1977 and 2001." *Am J Prev Med* **27**(3): 205-10.

Niemeier, H. et al. (2006). "Fast food consumption and breakfast skipping: predictors of weight gain from adolescence to adulthood in a nationally representative sample." *J Adolesc Health* **39**(6): 842-9.

Niemeier, H. et al. (2006). "Fast food consumption and breakfast skipping: Predictors of weight gain from adolescence to adulthood in a nationally representative sample." *Journal of Adolescent Health* **39**(6): 842-9.

Nies, M. et al. (1999). African American women's experiences with physical activity in their daily lives. *Public Health Nurs* **16**:23-31.

Noar, S. (2005-2006). "A health educator's guide to theories of health behavior." *Policy, Theory, and Social Issues* **24**: 75-92.

Noar, S. et al. (2008). "Applying health behavior theory to multiple behavior change: Considerations and approaches." *Preventive Medicine* **46**: 275-280.

Nord, M. et al. (2009). Household food security in the United States, 2008. *Economic Research Report No. (ERR-83)*, US Deptartment of Agriculture.

Novotny, R. et al. (2009). US acculturation, food intake, and obesity among Asian-Pacific hotel workers. *J Am Diet Assoc* **109**:1712-1718.

Nowjack-Raymer, R. and Sheiham, A. (2007). Numbers of natural teeth, diet, and nutritional status in US adults. *J Dent Res* **86**:1171-1175.

O'Dougherty, M. et al. (2008). Barriers and motivators for strength training among women of color and Caucasian women. *Women & Health* **47**(2) 41-62.

O'Dougherty, M. et al. (2006). "Nutrition labeling and value size pricing at fast-food restaurants: a consumer perspective." *Am J Health Promot* **20**(4): 247-50.

Ogden, C. (2009). "Disparities in obesity prevalence in the United States: black women at risk." *Am J Clin Nutr* **89**(4): 1001-2.

Ogden, C. et al. (2006). "Prevalence of Overweight and Obesity in the United States, 1999-2004." *JAMA* **295**(13): 1549-1555.

Ogden, C. et al. (2007). "Obesity among adults in the United States—no statistically significant change since 2003-2004." *NCHS Data Brief* **Nov**(1): 1-8.

Ogden, C. et al. (2010). "Prevalence of high body mass index in US children and adolescents, 2007-2008." *Jama* **303**(3): 242-9.

Oh, S. W., S. A. Shin, et al. (2004). "Cut-off point of BMI and obesity-related comorbidities and mortality in middle-aged Koreans." *Obes Res* **12**(12): 2031-40.

Okasha, M. et al. (2002). "Body mass index in young adulthood and cancer mortality: a retrospective cohort study." *J Epidemiol Community Health* **56**(10): 780-4.

Okosun, I. et al. (2001). "Abdominal obesity defined as a larger than expected waist girth is associated with racial/ethnic differences in risk of hypertension." *J Hum Hypertens* **15**(5): 307-12.

Olshansky, S. et al. (2005). "A potential decline in life expectancy in the United States in the 21st century." *N Engl J Med* **352**(11): 1138-45.

Ortega, R. et al. (1996). "Associations between obesity, breakfast time food habits and intake of energy and nutrients in a group of elderly Madrid residents." *J Am Coll Nutr* **15**(1): 65-72.

Otani, T. et al. (2005). "Body mass index, body height, and subsequent risk of colorectal cancer in middle-aged and elderly Japanese men and women: Japan public health center-based prospective study." *Cancer Causes Control* **16**(7): 839-50.

Paeratakul, S. et al. (2003). "Fast-food consumption among US adults and children: dietary and nutrient intake profile." *J Am Diet Assoc* **103**(10): 1332-8.

Papas, M. et al. (2007). "The built environment and obesity." *Epidemiol Rev* **29**: 129-43.

Patrick, H. and Nicklas, T. (2005). A review of family and social determinants of children's eating patterns and diet quality. *Journal of the American College of Nutrition* **24** (2): 83-92.

Patterson, R. et al. (2001). "Is there a consumer backlash against the diet and health message?" *J Am Diet Assoc* **101**(1): 37-41.

Pawlak, R. and Colby, S. (2009). Benefits, barriers, self-efficacy and knowledge regarding healthy foods; perception of African Americans living in eastern North Carolina. *Nutr Research and Practice* **3**:56-63.

Pelletier, A. et al. (2004). "Patients' understanding and use of snack food package nutrition labels." *J Am Board Fam Pract* **17**(5): 319-23.

Pereira, M. et al. (2005). "Fast-food habits, weight gain, and insulin resistance (the CARDIA study): 15-year prospective analysis." *Lancet* **365**(9453): 36-42.

Perez-Escamilla, R. and Putnik, P. (2007). "The role of acculturation in nutrition, lifestyle, and incidence of type 2 diabetes among Latinos." *J Nutrition* **137**: 860-70.

Pérez-Escamilla, R. et al. (2002). Translating knowledge into community nutrition programs: Lessons learned from the Connecticut Family Nutrition Program for Infants, Toddlers, and Children. *Recent Research Developments in Nutrition* **5**: 69–90.

Pérez-Escamilla, R. and Haldeman, L. (2002). Food label use modifies association of income with dietary quality. *J Nutr* **132**(4):768-72.

Pérez-Escamilla, R. et al. (2000). Marketing nutrition among urban Latinos: the SALUD! campaign. *J Am Diet Assoc* **100**(6):698-701.

Perrin, A. et al. (2002). "Ten-year trends of dietary intake in a middle-aged French population: relationship with educational level." *Eur J Clin Nutr* **56**(5): 393-401.

Peters, R. et al. (2006). African American culture and hypertension prevention. *Western J of Nursing Research*. **28**(7):831-854.

Petty, R. and Wegener, D. (1999). The Elaboration Likelihood Model: Current Status and Controversies. *Dual Process Theories in Social Psychology*. S. Chaiken and Y. Trope. New York, Guilford Press: 41–72.

Pierce, J. and Wardle, J. (1997). "Cause and effect beliefs and self-esteem of overweight children." *J Child Psychol Psychiatry* **38**(6): 645-50.

Pine, D. et al. (2001). "The association between childhood depression and adulthood body mass index." *Pediatrics* **107**(5): 1049-56.

Plescia, M. and Groblewski, M. (2004). A community-oriented primary care demonstration project: refining interventions for cardiovascular disease and diabetes. *Ann Fam Med* **2**:103-109.

Plescia, M. and Groblewski, M. (2004). "A community-oriented primary care demonstration project: refining interventions for cardiovascular disease and diabetes." *Ann Fam Med* **2**(2): 103-9.

Popkin, B. et al. Environmental influences on food choice, physical activity and energy balance. *Physiology and Behavior*. 2005;86:603-613.

Popkin, B. and Gordon-Larsen, P. The nutrition transition: worldwide obesity dynamics and their determinants. *Int J Obes*. 2004;28:S2-S9.

Popkin, B. and Udry, R. (1998). "Adolescent obesity increases significantly in second and third generation U.S. immigrants: The National Longitudinal Sutdy of Adolescent Health." *J Nutrition* **128**: 701-706.

Popkin, B. (2009). "What can public health nutritionists do to curb the epidemic of nutrition-related noncommunicable disease?" *Nutrition Reviews* **67**(s1): S79-S82.

Porter, J. et al. Psychosocial factors and perspectives on weight gain and barriers to weight loss among adolescents enrolled in obesity treatment. *J Clin Psychol Med Setting*. Online 2010.

Powell, L. and Chaloupka, F. (2009). "Food prices and obesity: evidence and policy implications for taxes and subsidies." *Milbank Q* **87**(1): 229-57.

Prentice, A. and Jebb, S. (2003). "Fast foods, energy density and obesity: a possible mechanistic link." *Obes Rev* **4**(4): 187-94.

Prevalence of overweight, obesity and extreme obesity among adults: United States, trends 1976-80 through 2005-2006. *Health E-Stats* 1-4.

Prochaska, J. et al. Eds. (2008). *The transtheoretical model and stages of change*. Health Behavior and Health Educ. Theory, Research, and Practice. San Francisco, Jossey-Bass.

Puhl, R. and Brownell, K. (2001). "Bias, discrimination, and obesity." *Obes Res* **9**(12): 788-805.

Puhl, R. and Heuer, C. (2009). "The stigma of obesity: a review and update." *Obesity (Silver Spring)* **17**(5): 941-64.

Puhl, R. and Heuer, C. (2010). "Obesity stigma: important considerations for public health." *Am J Public Health:* AJPH.2009.159491.

Puhl, R. and Brownell, K. (2006). "Confronting and coping with weight stigma: an investigation of overweight and obese adults." *Obesity (Silver Spring)* **14**(10): 1802-15.

Racette, S. et al. (2006). "Abdominal adiposity is a stronger predictor of insulin resistance than fitness among 50-95 year olds." *Diabetes Care* **29**(3): 673-8.

Raguso, C. et al. (1995). "Lipid and carbohydrate metabolism in IDDM during moderate and intense exercise." *Diabetes* **44**(9): 1066-74.

Rambeloson, Z. et al. (2008). "Linear programming can help identify practical solutions to improve the nutritional quality of food aid." *Public Health Nutr* **11**(4): 395-404.

Raynor, H. et al. (2002). "A cost-analysis of adopting a healthful diet in a family-based obesity treatment program." *J Am Diet Assoc* **102**(5): 645-56.

Reger, B. et al. (1998). 1% or less: a community-based nutrition campaign. *Public Health Rep* **113**(5):410-9.

Reid, D. and Hendricks, S. (1994). "Consumer understanding and use of fat and cholesterol information on food labels." *Can J Public Health* **85**(5): 334-7.

Reid, I. et al. (1992). "Fat mass is an important determinant of whole body bone density in premenopausal women but not in men." *J Clin Endocrinol Metab* **75**(3): 779-82.

Reid, I. et al. (1992). "Determinants of total body and regional bone mineral density in normal postmenopausal women—a key role for fat mass." *J Clin Endocrinol Metab* **75**(1): 45-51.

Renalds, A. et al. (2010). "A systematic review of built environment and health." *Fam Community Health* **33**(1): 68-78.

Resnicow, K. and Vaughan, R. (2006). "A chaotic view of behavior change: A quantum leap for health promotion." *International Journal of Behavioral Nutrition and Physical Activity* **3**: 25-30.

Rexrode, K. et al. (1997). "A prospective study of body mass index, weight change, and risk of stroke in women." *Jama* **277**(19): 1539-45.

Reyes-Ortiz C. et al. (2009). Neighborhood ethnic composition and diet among Mexican-Americans. *Public Health Nutrition.* **12**(12):2293-2301.

Ricciuto, L. and Tarasuk, V. (2007). "An examination of income-related disparities in the nutritional quality of food selections among Canadian households from 1986-2001." *Social Science & Medicine* **64**(1): 186-198.

Ricciuto, L. et al. (2005). "The relationship between price, amounts of saturated and trans fats, and nutrient content claims on margarines and oils." *Can J Diet Pract Res* **66**(4): 252-5.

Rimer, B. Ed. (2008). *Models of individual health behaviors.* Health Behavior and Health Education. Theory, Research, and Practice. San Francisco, Jossey-Bass.

Roberts, R. et al. (2003). "Prospective association between obesity and depression: evidence from the Alameda County Study." *Int J Obes Relat Metab Disord* **27**(4): 514-21.

Robinson, W. et al. (2009). "The female-male disparity in obesity prevalence among black American young adults: contributions of sociodemographic characteristics of the childhood family." *Am J Clin Nutr* **89**(4): 1204-12.

Rodriguez, C. et al. (2001). "Body mass index, height, and prostate cancer mortality in two large cohorts of adult men in the United States." *Cancer Epidemiol Biomarkers Prev* **10**(4): 345-53.

Rodriguez, C. et al. (2002). "Body mass index, height, and the risk of ovarian cancer mortality in a prospective cohort of postmenopausal women." *Cancer Epidemiol Biomarkers Prev* **11**(9): 822-8.

Rolls, B. et al. (2002). Portion size of food affects energy intake in normal-weight and overweight men and women. *Am J Clin Nutr* **76**: 1207-13.

Romero-Gwynn, E. et al. (1993). "Dietary acculturation among Latinos of Mexican descent." *Nutrition Today* **July/August**: 6-12.

Rose, D. and Richards, R. (2004). "Food store access and household fruit and vegetable use among participants in the US Food Stamp Program." *Public Health Nutr* **7**(8): 1081-8.

Rosenthal, A. et al. (2004). "Body fat distribution and risk of diabetes among Chinese women." *Int J Obes Relat Metab Disord* **28**(4): 594-9.

Rothman, A. (2004). ""Is there nothing more practical than a good theory?" Why innovations and advances in health behavior change will arise if interventions are used to test and refine theory." *International Journal of Behavioral Nutrition and Physical Activity* **1**: 11-17.

Roux, C. et al. (1999). "Comportement alimentaire - Food attitudes and behaviours of low-income populations." *Cahiers de nutrition et de diÈtÈtique.* **34**(6): 378.

Rowlands, J. and Hoadley, J (2006). "FDA perspectives on health claims for food labels." *Toxicology* **221**(1): 35-43.

Rutt, C. and Coleman, K. (2005). Examining the relationships among built environment, physical activity, and body mass index in El Paso, TX. *Prev Med* **40**:831-841.

Salbe, A. et al. (2002). "Assessing risk factors for obesity between childhood and adolescence: I. Birth weight, childhood adiposity, parental obesity, insulin, and leptin." *Pediatrics* **110**(2 Pt 1): 299-306.

Salbe, A. et al. (2002). "Assessing risk factors for obesity between childhood and adolescence: II. Energy metabolism and physical activity." *Pediatrics* **110**(2 Pt 1): 307-14.

Sallis, J. (2000). Age-related decline in physical activity: a synthesis of human an animal studies. *Med Sci Sports Exerc* **32**:1598-600.

Sallis, J. et al., Eds. (2008). *Ecological Models of Health Behavior.* Health Behavior and Health Educ. Theory, Research, and Practice. San Francisco, Jossey-Bass.

Sampson, A. et al. (1995). "The nutritional impact of breakfast consumption on the diets of inner-city African-American elementary school children." *J Natl Med Assoc* **87**(3): 195-202.

Sandoval, W. et al. (1994). "Stages of change: A model for nutrition counseling." *Topics in Clinical Nutrition* **9**: 64-69.

Sartorio, A. et al. (2005). "Gender-related changes in body composition, muscle strength and power output after a short-term multidisciplinary weight loss intervention in morbid obesity." *J Endocrinol Invest* **28**(6): 494-501.

Satia, J. et al. (2005). "Food nutrition label use is associated with demographic, behavioral, and psychosocial factors and dietary intake among African Americans in North Carolina." *J Am Diet Assoc* **105**(3): 392-402; discussion 402-3.

Satia, J. et al. (2000). "Use of qualitative methods to study diet, acculturation, and health in Chinese-American women." *J Am Diet Assoc* **100**(8): 934-40.

Satia-Abouta, J. et al. (2002). "Dietary acculturation: applications to nutrition research and dietetics." *J Am Diet Assoc* **102**: 1105-1118.

Sattar, N. et al. (1998). "Associations of indices of adiposity with atherogenic lipoprotein subfractions." *Int J Obes Relat Metab Disord* **22**(5): 432-9.

Savage, J. et al. (2009). "Dieting, restraint, and disinhibition predict women's weight change over 6 y." *Am J Clin Nutr* **90**(1): 33-40.

Scharf, M. et al. (2005). "Sibling relationships in emerging adulthood and in adolescence." *Journal of Adolescent Research* **20**(1): 64-90.

Scharff, D. et al. (1999). Factors associated with physical activity in women across the life span: implications for program development. *Women Health* **29**:115-34.

Schlundt, D. et al. (1992). "The role of breakfast in the treatment of obesity: a randomized clinical trial." *Am J Clin Nutr* **55**(3): 645-51.

Schulter, G. and Lee, C. (1999). Changing food consumption patterns: their effect on the U.S. food system, 1972-92. *Food Review* **22**(1):35-38.

Schuz, B. et al. (2009). "Predicting transitions from preintentional, intentional and actional stages of change." *Health Education Research* **24**: 64-75.

Schwartz, M. et al. (2003). "Weight bias among health professionals specializing in obesity." *Obes Res* **11**(9): 1033-9.

Schwartz, M. and Brownell, K. (2007). Actions necessary to prevent childhood obesity: creating the climate for change. *J Law Med Ethics* **35**(1):78-89.

Schwartzer, R. (2001). "Social-Cognitive Factors in Changing Health-Related Behaviors." *Current Directions in Psychological Science* **10**: 47-51.

Segal, K. et al. (1988). "Lean body mass estimation by bioelectrical impedance analysis: a four-site cross-validation study." *Am J Clin Nutr* **47**(1): 7-14.

Serdula, M. et al. (1993). "Do obese children become obese adults? A review of the literature." *Preventive Medicine* **22**: 167-177.

Sharkey, J. and Horel, S. (2008). Neighborhood socioeconomic deprivation and minority composition are associated with better potential spatial access to the ground-truthed food environment in a large rural area. *J. Nutr* **138**:620-627.

Shepherd, J. et al. (2006). Young people and healthy eating: a systematic review of research on barriers and facilitators. *Health Educ Res* **21**:239-257.

Siega-Riz, A. et al. (1998). "Three squares or mostly snacks—what do teens really eat? A sociodemographic study of meal patterns." *J Adolesc Health* **22**(1): 29-36.

Simon, P. et al. (2008). Proximity of fast-food restaurants to schools: Do neighborhood income and type of school matter? *Preventive Medicine* **47**(3):284-288.

Sisson, S. et al. (2009). "Profiles of sedentary behavior in children and adolescents: the US National Heal

Siwik, V. and Senf, J. (2006). Food cravings, ethnicity and other factors related to eating out. *J Am Clin Nutr* **25**(5): 382-388.

Smeets, T. et al. (2007). "Effects of Tailored Feedback on Multiple Health Behaviors." *Annals of Behavioral Medicine* **33**: 117–123.

Smith, C. and Morton, L. (2009). Rural food deserts: low-income perspectives on food access in Minnesota and Iowa. *J Nutr Educ Behav* **41**:176-187.

Sneed, J. and Burkhalter, J. (1991). "Marketing nutrition in restaurants: a survey of current practices and attitudes." *J Am Diet Assoc* **91**(4): 459-62.

Sobal, J. and Stunkard, A. (1989). "Socioeconomic status and obesity: a review of the literature." *Psychological Bulletin* **105**(2): 260-75.

Sonneville, K. et al. (2009). Economic and other barriers to adopting recommendations to prevent childhood obesity: results of a focus group study with parents. *BMC Pediatrics.* **81** (9).

Spear, B. (2002). Adolescent growth and development. *J Am Diet Assoc* **102**:S23-S29.

Sproul, A. et al. (2003). "Does point-of-purchase nutrition labeling influence meal selections? A test in an Army cafeteria." *Mil Med* **168**(7): 556-60.

St Jeor, S. et al. (1997). "A classification system to evaluate weight maintainers, gainers, and losers." *J Am Diet Assoc* **97**(5): 481-8.

Steffen, L. et al. (2009). "Overweight in children and adolescents associated with TV viewing and parental weight: Project HeartBeat!" *Am J Prev Med* **37**(1 Suppl): S50-5.

Stender, S. et al. (1993). "Cholesterol-lowering diets may increase the food costs for Danish children. A cross-sectional study of food costs for Danish children with and without familial hypercholesterolaemia." *Eur J Clin Nutr* **47**(11): 776-86.

Stevens, J. et al. (2002). "Fitness and fatness as predictors of mortality from all causes and from cardiovascular disease in men and women in the Lipid Research Clinics Study." *Am. J. Epidemiol.* **156**(9): 832-841.

Stewart, H. et al. (2006). "Let's eat out Americans weigh taste, convenience and nutrition." from http://purl.access.gpo.gov/GPO/LPS76124.

Steyn, N. et al. (2004). "Diet, nutrition and the prevention of type 2 diabetes."*Public Health Nutr* **7**(1A): 147-65.

Stopka, T. (2002). An innovative community-based approach to encourage breastfeeding among Hispanic/Latino women. *J Am Diet Assoc* **102**(6):766-7.

Story, M. and Neumark-Sztainer, D. (2005). "A perspective on family meals: Do they matter?" *Nutrition Today* **40**(6): 261-266.

Story, M. and Alton, I. (1996). "Adolescent nutrition: Current trends and critical issues." *Topics in Clinical Nutrition* **11**(3): 56-69.

Story, M. and Resnick, M. (1986). "Adolescents' views on food and nutrition." *Journal of Nutrition Education* **18**(4): 188-192.

Story, M. et al. (2002). "Individual and environmental influences on adolescent eating behaviors." *J Am Diet Assoc* **102**(3 Suppl): S40 51.

Strauss, R. and Knight J. (1999). "Influence of the home environment on the development of obesity in children." *Pediatrics* **103**(6): e85.

Strong, K. et al. (2008). Weight gain prevention: identifying theory-based targets for health behavior change in young adults. *J Am Diet Assoc* **108**:1708-1715.

Stunkard, A. and Messick, S. (1985). "The three-factor eating questionnaire to measure dietary restraint, disinhibition and hunger." *J Psychosom Res* **29**(1): 71-83.

Sturm, R. et al. (2004). "Increasing obesity rates and disability trends." *Health Aff (Millwood)* **23**(2): 199-205.

Summerbell, C. et al. (1996). "Relationship between feeding pattern and body mass index in 220 free-living people in four age groups." *Eur J Clin Nutr* **50**(8): 513-9.

Sundquist, J. and Winkleby, M. (2000). Country of birth, acculturation status and abdominal obesity in a nation sample of Mexican-American women and men. In *J Epidemiol* **29**:470-477.

Tanaka, S. et al. (2002). "Is adiposity at normal body weight relevant for cardiovascular disease risk?" *Int J Obes Relat Metab Disord* **26**(2): 176-83.

Tanasescu, M. et al. (2000) Biobehavioral factors are associated with obesity in Puerto Rican children. *J Nutr* **130**(7):1734-42.

Taras, H. and Gage, M. (1995). Advertised foods on children's television. *Arch Pediatr Adolesc Med* **149**(6):649-52.

Tarasuk, V. et al. (2007). "Low-income women's dietary intakes are sensitive to the depletion of household resources in one month." *Journal of Nutrition* **137**(8): 1980-1987.

Taylor, A. et al. (2010). "Comparison of the associations of body mass index and measures of central adiposity and fat mass with coronary heart disease, diabetes, and all-cause mortality: a study using data from 4 UK cohorts." *Am J Clin Nutr:* ajcn.2009.28757.

Taylor, E. et al. (2005). "Obesity, weight gain, and the risk of kidney stones." *Jama* **293**(4): 455-62.

Terracciano, A.. et al. (2009). "Facets of Personality Linked to Underweight and Overweight." *Psychosomatic Medicine* **71**(6): 682-689.

Thornton, A. et al. (1995). "Parent-child relationships during the transition to adulthood." *Journal of Family Issues* **16**: 538-564.

Thorpe, K. et al. (2004). "The impact of obesity on rising medical spending." *Health Aff (Millwood)* **Suppl Web Exclusives**: W4-480-6.

Timperio, A.. et al. (2010). "Neighbourhood physical activity environments and adiposity in children and mothers: a three-year longitudinal study." *Int J Behav Nutr Phys Act* 7(1): 18.

Torres, S. and Nowson, C. (2007). "Relationship between stress, eating behavior, and obesity." *Nutrition* 23(11-12): 887-94.

Townsend, M. et al.(2009). "Low energy-dense diets are more costly for low-income women in California." *American Journal of Clinical Nutrition* **In Press**.

Turrell, G. et al. (2010). "Neighborhood disadvantage and physical activity: baseline results from the HABITAT multilevel longitudinal study." *Ann Epidemiol* **20**(3): 171-81.

Tylor, E. (1924). Primitive Culture. New York, NY, Brentano's.

U.S. Department of Health and Human Services (2000). Health Communication. *Healthy People 2010, Understanding and Improving Health.* Washington, DC, U.S. Government Printing Office.

United States. Dept. of, H. and S. Human (2000). *Healthy People 2010.* Washington, D.C., The Dept.

Ver Ploeg, M.et al. (2009). Access to affordable and nutritious food measuring and understanding food deserts and their consequences: report to Congress.

Victor, L. et al. (2009). Fulgoni III, Debra R. Keast, Adam Drewnowski Development and Validation of the Nutrient-Rich Foods Index: A Tool to Measure Nutritional Quality of Foods. *Journal of Nutrition* **139**:1-6.

Videon, T. and. Manning, C. (2003). "Influences on adolescent eating patterns: The importance of family meals." *Journal of Adolescent Health* **32**: 365-373.

Vozoris, N. et al. (2002). "The affordability of a nutritious diet for households on welfare in Toronto." *Canadian Journal of Public Health-Revue Canadienne De Sante Publique* **93**(1): 36-40.

Wallinga, D. et al. (2009). "Considering the Contribution of US Agricultural Policy to the Obesity Epidemic: Overview and Opportunities." *Journal of Hunger & Environmental Nutrition* **4**(1): 3-19.

Walsh, J. et al. (2009). Using focus groups to identify factors affecting healthy weight maintenance in college men. *Nutrition Research.* 29:371-378.

Wansink, B. et al. (2009). "Is this a meal or snack?" Situational cues that drive perceptions. *Appetite* **54**(1):214-218.

Wansink, B. (2004) Environmental factors that increase the food intake and consumption volume of unknowing customers. *Annual Review of Nutrition* **24**:455-79.

Wardle, J. et al. (2000). "Nutrition knowledge and food intake." *Appetite* **34**(3): 269-275.

Warnick, E. et al. (2004). Social marketing improved the use of multivitamin and mineral supplements among resource-poor women in Bolivia. *J Nutr Educ Behav* **36**(6):290-7.

Webber, C. et al. (2010). Shopping for fruits and vegetables. Food and retail qualities of importance to low-income households at the grocery store. *Appetite* **54**:297-303.

Webber, L. et al. (1986). "Transitions of cardiovascular risk from adolescence to young adulthood—the Bogalusa Heart Study: II. Alterations in anthropometric blood pressure and serum lipoprotein variables." *Journal of Chronic Diseases* **39**(2): 91-103.

Weinstein, N. et al. (1998). "Stage Theories of Health Behavior: Conceptual and Methodological Issues." *Health Psychology* **17**: 290-299.

Weinstein, N. et al., Eds. (2008). *The precaution adoption process model.* Health Behavior and Health Educ. Theory, Research, and Practice. San Francisco, Jossey-Bass.

Weintraub, J. et al. (2002). "A prospective study of the relationship between body mass index and cataract extraction among US women and men." *Int J Obes Relat Metab Disord* **26**(12): 1588-95.

Wen, L. et al. (2004). Family support and diet barriers among older Hispanic adults with type 2 diabetes. *Fam Med* **36**(6):423-30.

West and et al. (1999). "Food preparation practices influence nutrition." *California agriculture.* **53**(1): 29.

Whitaker, R. et al. (1998). "Early adiposity rebound and the risk of adult obesity." *Pediatrics* **101**(3): E5.

Wiecha, J. et al. (2006). When children eat what they watch. *Arch Pediatr Adolesc Med* **160**: 436-442.

Wiig-Dammann, K. and Smith, C. (2009). "Factors Affecting Low-income Women's Food Choices and the Perceived Impact of Dietary Intake and Socioeconomic Status on Their Health and Weight." *Journal of Nutrition Education and Behavior* **41**(4): 242-253.

Wilcox, S. et al. (2000). Determinants of leisure time physical activity in rural compared with urban older and ethnically diverse women in the United States. *Journal of Epidemiology and Community Health* **54**;9:667-672.

Wilde, P. (2009). "Self-regulation and the response to concerns about food and beverage marketing to children in the United States." *Nutr Rev* **67**(3): 155-66.

Wilde, P. and Llobrera, J. (2009). Using the Thrifty Food Plan to Asses the Cost of a Nutritious Diet. *Journal of Consumer Affairs.* **43**(2):p.274-304.

Williams, M. (2002). Nutrition for Health, Fitness and Sport. New York, McGraw-Hill.

Williamson, D. et al. (1995). "Association of body mass with dietary restraint and disinhibition." *Appetite* **25**(1): 31-41.

Wilsgaard, T., H. Schirmer, et al. (2000). "Impact of body weight on blood pressure with a focus on sex differences: the Tromso Study, 1986-1995." *Arch Intern Med* **160**(18): 2847-53.

Wilson, N. et al. (1999) Food ads on TV: a health hazard for children? *Aust N Z J Public Health 23(6):647-50.*

Wintre, M. and Yaffe, M. (2000). "First-year students' adjustment to university life as a funciton of relationships with parents." *Journal of Adolescent Research* **15**: 9-37.

Wolfe, W. and Campbell, C. (1993). "Food pattern, diet quality, and related characteristics of schoolchildren in New York State." *J Am Diet Assoc* **93**(11): 1280-4.

Wolfe, W. et al. (1994). "Overweight school children in New York State: prevalence and characteristics." *American Journal of Public Health* **84**(5): 807-13.

World Cancer Research Fund / American Institute for Cancer Research (2007). Food, Nutrition, Physical Activity and the Prevention of Cancer: a Global Perspective. AICR. Washington, DC.

World Health Organization (1998). Obesity: preventing and managing the global epidemic. Geneva, World Health Organization.

Xu, W. et al. (2005). "Effect of adiposity and fat distribution on endometrial cancer risk in Shanghai women." *Am J Epidemiol* **161**(10): 939-47.

Yancey, A. et al. (2009). A cross-sectional prevalence study of ethnically targeted and general audience outdoor obesity-related advertising. *Milbank Q* **87**(1):155-84.

Yanovski, J. et al. (2000). "A prospective study of holiday weight gain." *N Engl J Med* **342**(12): 861-7.

Yeh M. et al. (2008). Understanding barriers and facilitators of fruit and vegetable consumption among a diverse multi-ethnic population in the USA. *Health Promot Iat* **23**:42-51.

Yeh, W. et al. (2005). "Do centrally obese Chinese with normal BMI have increased risk of metabolic disorders?" *Int J Obes (Lond)* **29**(7): 818-25.

Young, L. and Nestle, M. (2002). "The contribution of expanding portion sizes to the US obesity epidemic." *Am J Public Health* **92**(2): 246-9.

Zagorsky, J. and Smith, P. (2009). "Does the U.S. Food Stamp Program contribute to adult weight gain?" *Econ Hum Biol* **7**(2): 246-58.

Zenk, S. et al. (2005). Fruit and vegetable intake in African Americans income an store characteristics. *Am J Prev Med* **29**:1-9.

Zhao, L. et al. (2008). "Correlation of obesity and osteoporosis: effect of fat mass on the determination of osteoporosis." *J Bone Miner Res* **23**(1): 17-29.

Zhu, S. et al. (2004). "Combination of BMI and Waist Circumference for Identifying Cardiovascular Risk Factors in Whites." *Obes Res* **12**(4): 633-45.

Zhu, S. et al. (2002). "Waist circumference and obesity-associated risk factors among whites in the third National Health and Nutrition Examination Survey: clinical action thresholds." *Am J Clin Nutr* **76**(4): 743-9.

Zhu, S. et al. (2003). "Percentage body fat ranges associated with metabolic syndrome risk: results based on the third National Health and Nutrition Examination Survey (1988-1994)." *Am J Clin Nutr* **78**(2): 228-35.

Zimmerman, F. and Bell, J. (2010). "Associations of television content type and obesity in children." *Am J Public Health* **100**(2): 334-40.

Zunft, H. et al. (1999). Perceived benefits and barriers to physical activity in a nationally representative sample in the European Union. *Public Health Nutr* **2**:153-160.